(Num)

EMERGENCY PHYSIOTHERAPY

For Churchill Livingstone:

Senior Commissioning Editor: Heidi Allen
Project Development Manager: Mairi McCubbin
Project Manager: Derek Robertson
Design Direction: Judith Wright
Illustrations Manager: Bruce Hogarth

EMERGENCY PHYSIOTHERAPY

Beverley Harden MSc MCSP

*Superintendent Physiotherapist, Southampton
University Hospital's Trust, Southampton, UK*

Foreword by

Jennifer A. Pryor MSc MBA FNZSP MCSP

Royal Brompton Hospital, London, UK

CHURCHILL
LIVINGSTONE

EDINBURGH LONDON NEW YORK OXFORD PHILADELPHIA
ST LOUIS SYDNEY TORONTO 2004

CHURCHILL LIVINGSTONE
An imprint of Elsevier Science Limited

First published 2004

ISBN 0 443 07301 5

British Library Cataloguing in Publication Data
A catalogue record for this book is available from the British Library

Library of Congress Cataloging in Publication Data
A catalog record for this book is available from the Library of Congress

Notice
Medical knowledge is constantly changing. Standard safety precautions must be
followed, but as new research and clinical experience broaden our knowledge, changes
in treatment and drug therapy may become necessary or appropriate. Readers are
advised to check the most current product information provided by the manufacturer
of each drug to be administered to verify the recommended dose, the method and
duration of administration, and contraindications. It is the responsibility of the
practitioner, relying on experience and knowledge of the patient, to determine dosages
and the best treatment for each individual patient. Neither the Publisher nor the editor
assumes any liability for any injury and/or damage to persons or property arising from
this publication.

The Publisher

The
publisher's
policy is to use
**paper manufactured
from sustainable forests**

Printed in China

Contents

12. Calls to the surgical unit *Valerie Ball* 157

Contributors

Alison Aldridge MCSP SRP
Lecturer in Physiotherapy, University of Southampton, Southampton, UK

Valerie Ball MSc MCSP
Clinical Physiotherapy Specialist, Staffordshire General Hospital, Stafford, UK

Sarah Boyce MCSP
Clinical Specialist Physiotherapist, University College Hospital, London, UK

Alison Carter MCSP
Superintendent Physiotherapist, Guy's and St Thomas's Hospitals Trust, London, UK

Lorraine Clapham MCSP
Superintendent Physiotherapist, Southampton General Hospital, Southampton, UK

Nell Clotworthy MSc MCSP
Clinical Specialist, Cardio-respiratory Physiotherapy, St George's Hospital, London, UK

Jane Cross MCSP
Senior Lecturer in Physiotherapy, University of East Anglia, Norwich, UK

Rachel Devlin MCSP
Clinical Specialist Physiotherapist, Southampton University Hospital's Trust, Southampton, UK

Elaine Dhouieb MCSP
Assistant Lead Physiotherapist, Royal Hospital for Sick Children, Edinburgh, UK

Alison Draper MCSP
Senior Lecturer in Physiotherapy, University of Liverpool, Liverpool, UK

Beverley Harden MSc MCSP
Superintendent Physiotherapist, Southampton University Hospital's Trust, Southampton, UK

Stephen Harden MA MB BS FRCS FRCR
Senior Radiology Registrar, Southampton University Hospital's Trust, Southampton, UK

Bernadette Henderson MSc MCSP
Superintendent Physiotherapist, Barnet Hospital; Honorary Lecturer, University College, London, UK

Hazel Horobin MA MSc MCSP
Senior Lecturer in Physiotherapy, Sheffield Hallam University, Sheffield, UK

Carole Jones MCSP
Superintendent Physiotherapist, University Hospital of Wales, Cardiff, UK

Sarah E. J. Keilty MSc MCSP
Consultant Physiotherapist, Acute Medicine and Critical Care Directorate, Guy's and St Thomas's NHS Trust, London, UK

Katharine Malhotra MCSP
Superintendent Physiotherapist, Royal Marsden Hospital, London, UK

Paul Ritson GradDipPhys MCSP
Clinical Specialist PICU Physiotherapist, Royal Liverpool Children's NHS Trust (Alder Hey), Liverpool, UK

Fiona E. Roberts BSc MCSP
Senior Lecturer in Physiotherapy, Sheffield Hallam University, Sheffield, UK

Sandy Thomas MEd MCSP Cert Ed Dip TP
Senior Lecturer in Physiotherapy, University of the West of England, Bristol, UK

Nicola Thompson MCSP
Superintendent Physiotherapist, Royal Marsden Hospital, London, UK

Ruth Wakeman BSc (Hons) MCSP
Senior 1 Paediatric Physiotherapist, Royal Brompton Hospital, London, UK

Foreword

Most of us can recall our first on calls: the mixed emotions of excitement, responsibility and anxiety. We try to, but cannot possibly, remember everything that is in our cardiorespiratory textbook. We hope that our assessment of the patient will accurately identify the patient's problems and that our treatment, and adaptation of our treatment dependent on the outcome, will be effective. With experience we can speed up the clinical reasoning process, but the same principles apply and these principles should be evidence based.

All too often we denigrate the evidence that does exist in support of many of the techniques used in cardiorespiratory physiotherapy. Evidence-based practice is the integration of individual clinical expertise and the best external evidence (Sackett et al 1996). In physiotherapy, clinical expertise – 'the proficiency and judgment that individual clinicians acquire through clinical experience and clinical practice' – is an important part of our current evidence. There will always be unanswered questions as each piece of research produces more research questions.

Emergency Physiotherapy – an On-Call Survival Guide is evidence based where possible. The text complements the emergency respiratory on-call working guidance for physiotherapists developed by the Association of Chartered Physiotherapists in Respiratory Care (ACPRC) and the Chartered Society of Physiotherapy (CSP) (ACPRC & CSP 2002). Beverley Harden and her team of authors are to be commended on their achievement of a pocket-sized, ready-reference text to accompany the clinical physiotherapist working with people with cardiorespiratory problems – adults and children.

Jennifer Pryor, 2004

References

ACPRC, CSP (2002) Emergency respiratory on call working: guidance for physiotherapists. (Ref: PA53). London: Chartered Society of Physiotherapy.

Sackett DL, Rosenberg WM, Gray JA et al (1996) Evidence based medicine: what it is and what it isn't. BMJ 312 (7023): 71–72.

Preface

Treating respiratory patients out of hours can be a daunting experience for most physiotherapists for several reasons. The patient is unwell; you may need to act quickly in an unfamiliar environment; you generally do not have on-site senior physiotherapy support; and you may not regularly work with respiratory patients.

This book is designed to support you in this situation. It aims to support your learning in the form of a comprehensive, yet concise, account of the information needed by on-call physiotherapists.

This book should not be considered a core textbook: it is a vehicle to bring key information, in an accessible format, into the work environment, to facilitate safe and effective physiotherapy. It aims to refer the reader on to the appropriate evidence-based learning resources.

Respiratory care is a core physiotherapy skill. As a professional it is your responsibility to maintain and update your skills, supported by your employer, and to make yourself aware of, and adhere to, your local hospital policies regarding the treatment of cardiorespiratory patients. It may have been a significant time since you completed your respiratory training; thus regular self-directed learning alongside practical training and assessment of competence are all integral parts of maintaining and developing these skills and your confidence.

This book will also support students on cardiorespiratory clinical placements and staff undertaking a period of adaptation or returning to work. The intention, in writing the book, was to harness the knowledge of the senior clinicians and encapsulate this on paper: to create a 'senior physiotherapist in your pocket'. Thank you to the authors and reviewers who have taken so much time and trouble to achieve this near-impossible task!

How to Use this Book
This book is designed to complement on-call training. Every patient scenario is different and you must respond accordingly. The book only gives ideas for treatment, not recipes. It is essential that you assess patients fully and treat them appropriately.

Do not be put off by:

- elements of repetition – this is essential if the information is to be accessible to the reader
- the fact that you may not have access to some of the equipment or knowledge referred to in the book. In each instance several treatment options are examined. Use the techniques available to you and that you feel confident with.

The book will help to make on call a learning experience. Use Chapters 19 and 20 to help guide this process, to ensure that your knowledge and skills base continue to develop.

Beverley Harden
Southampton, 2004

Acknowledgements

Sincere thanks to everyone who has supported this work by: writing chapters; reading chapters; reviewing chapters; rereading chapters; and sharing their specialist knowledge. Special thanks to Jennifer Pryor, Alex Hough, Mary Ann Broad, Kim Ainsworth and Janet Webber, who offered their continued support and expertise throughout the editing of the book.

Thank you also to Elsevier Science who have supported the concept of this book from its first beginnings.

Above all thanks to Stephen and James for patiently putting up with the time lost to the book, and without whose support it would never have become a reality.

CHAPTER 1 On call preparation

Carole Jones

Respiratory physiotherapy on call presents each clinician with a challenging work environment. This chapter suggests how you can prepare for on call and learn from your experiences to guide your continuing professional development.

PREPARATION

On Call Policy/Procedure
You should request a copy of the departmental policy. Read this carefully; it will include valuable information on the operational aspects of the on call service, such as the:

- On call period, e.g. 5 p.m.–9 a.m. It is essential that you are free to respond to a call at any time within that on call period.
- Referral criteria. There should be clear guidelines for medical staff about the type of patient who should be referred to the on call service.
- Response time. If your travel time exceeds the agreed response time you will need to stay in hospital accommodation. Discuss this with the senior respiratory physiotherapist, who will be able to help you access an on call room if appropriate.
- Payment.
- Time in lieu arrangements.
- Organization of the rota.
- Health and safety issues, e.g.:
  a. parking and accessing the department at night, working alone, the availability of personal alarms, taxis, etc.
  b. infection control.

Infection Control
- Before you are on call, read your organization's infection control policy. Remember that policies vary between organizations and over time. Be aware of your own vaccination record and how

additional factors such as your own early pregnancy might influence your risk assessment.

- Sick patients may have a number of drips and drains producing risk of contact with body fluids and exposure to blood-borne pathogens. Make sure you know what is expected of universal precautions and where in your place of work you can access the protective clothing and equipment required. Be aware of what to do in the event of a needlestick injury or splash incident to the eyes or mouth.

- Sick patients will have a reduced capacity to overcome further infection and may have numerous access points (drips/drains/catheters) for infection to be introduced. Exercise care for all patients as directed by your policy. Be prepared to check for additional instructions if you are called to a patient being nursed in isolation.

- Physiotherapy techniques can increase the quantity of respiratory pathogens exhaled into room air. Find out from your policy what infections require special respiratory precautions and how you are expected to manage them, for example TB.

Remember:
If you are unsure of the precautions you should take, ask before commencing treatment.

Assessment of Your Learning Needs

There will be an opportunity to formally assess your knowledge and skills with a senior clinician. This will ensure that you have a basic level of competence prior to commencing on call. Use this opportunity to identify your individual training needs and develop an action plan with your senior. You are expected to have learning needs; qualification as a physiotherapist does not mean that you are fully competent or that you feel confident to work on call.

Clinical Experience Within Different Clinical Specialties

(e.g. Paediatrics, Neurosurgery, Intensive Care, Medicine, etc.)
Aim to familiarize yourself with the following:

- The geography of the hospital and ward environments.
- The treatment guidelines/protocols for the specialities within your hospital.

- Specific limitations/contraindications to treatment.
- The clinical workload. You can do this by working alongside a mentor:
  a. observe and discuss assessment
  b. discuss clinical reasoning/problem solving
  c. observe the application of treatment modalities and their evaluation
  d. assess and treat patients under the guidance of your mentor, discuss your clinical reasoning, choice of treatment options and evaluation/modification of treatment.
- The location of equipment:
  a. Where is the respiratory equipment (e.g. IPPB) stored?
  b. How will you access it at night?
  Some equipment (e.g. suction catheters, humidification, etc.) may be stored on the ward. Familiarize yourself with the location.
- Assembly of respiratory equipment. Assemble equipment (e.g. IPPB circuits, humidification circuits, etc.) under supervision as systems will vary from trust to trust.
- How to access patient information.

Lectures/In-Service Training
Alongside your individualized learning in the clinical environment each department should have access to an ongoing learning process involving workshops and lectures designed to update and consolidate staff on key respiratory topics.

Shadow On Call
Request the opportunity to shadow a senior colleague on call. Use this opportunity to:

- Observe the on call procedure, e.g. contacting the switch board, travelling, parking, attending the call and discussing the case, recording attendance, claiming payment, etc.
- As your confidence builds, take the lead with the support and guidance of your mentor. You may now feel confident with their support on the phone.
- Discuss your clinical reasoning, proposed treatment plan or any problems you have encountered.

With a comprehensive induction programme and self-directed learning, your confidence will build. On call will become much less daunting when you know you have the support and guidance of your senior staff.

THE DAY OF YOUR ON CALL

There are a number of points to remember:

- Was anybody called out on the previous night? If so, are further call outs to this patient required? Has the patient improved with treatment through the course of the day?
- Review/treat the patient with the appropriate clinician or your mentor.
- Liaise with colleagues across the other specialities to identify patients who may require on call. Take the opportunity before the end of the day to review the patient with senior staff.
- Prioritize and discuss your own caseload with your senior ensuring cover for the next day; this will be determined by your local European Working Time Directive agreement.
- Before leaving work, contact the hospital switchboard to advise them on a point of contact, your pager and/or telephone number. Give both mobile and landline numbers.

  Remember to take with you:
  a. an agreed (confidential) list of contact numbers for the senior clinicians
  b. a copy of the on call referral criteria
  c. a list of questions to ask if called; this will allow you to remain focused despite any underlying panic!
  d. your uniform, stethoscope, pager or phone.

THE TELEPHONE CALL

Questions to Ask
- What is the patient's name?
- Does the patient meet the criteria for on call referral?
- Which ward is the patient on and how to find it?
- To whom are you speaking? Has the doctor referred the patient? If not, has the patient had a medical review? Some policies do accept referral from nursing staff, so be aware of your local policy.
- Ascertain a brief history of the patient's condition. What were they admitted with?
- Has the patient already been referred to physiotherapy? If so, when did the patient last receive treatment? You will need to retrieve the case notes.
- How has the patient deteriorated? Has it been sudden or gradual?

- What appears to be the problem?
- Has the patient had blood gases taken and/or a chest X-ray?
- What measures have the medical team or nurses taken to improve the patient's condition, for example suction or oxygen therapy?
- How did the patient respond?

Think ahead. You only have a brief outline of the patient's condition. Decide what further information you will need on your arrival to complete a full assessment. The nursing staff can liaise with the medical staff and may be able to collect this information and have it ready for you on your arrival.

ADVICE TO CONSIDER WHILE ON THE PHONE

- Is the patient on humidified oxygen?
- Has the patient been prescribed bronchodilators? If so, request a dose be given as you travel in. If the patient is having difficulty clearing thick secretions, can nebulized saline be prescribed and given?
- Can the patient's oxygen be increased? (Remember this should be agreed with the doctor.)
- You may be able to advise on positioning to reduce work of breathing or improve V/Q match.
- Is pain adequately controlled, e.g. is the patient able to move, cough, etc.? If not, this will need to be better managed prior to your arrival.
- Is the patient going to have more tests, etc.? If so, when will you be able to see the patient?

As you travel in you will have begun to piece together the information and have some idea of the treatment modalities you may use. For example, do you need to pick up equipment such as IPPB on your way to the ward?

EFFECTIVE COMMUNICATION IN THE ON CALL SETTING

General Communication With the Medical/Nursing Staff

Faced by the acutely unwell patient, you may need to act quickly to prevent further deterioration. Other members of the team will be familiar with the patient and can give you valuable information for your assessment:

- Speak to the nurse responsible for the patient to gain a more in-depth assessment of the patient's history and recent deterioration.

- Did any of the advice you gave improve the patient's condition or has the patient continued to deteriorate since they called you?
- Do you need the nurse to assist you with your assessment or treatment.
- Contact the doctor if required.
- Document your assessment/treatment/outcome and when the patient will next be reviewed in the medical notes.

Communication With the Patient/Relatives

- Explain your role to the patient and how you can help. This can reduce anxiety and distress.
- If relatives are present explain your role and how you are going to help. Ask the patient whether or not they would like the relatives present during treatment.
- Relatives may, however, express concern about the proposed treatment, despite a full explanation. In this situation, you must seek the guidance of the doctor, who may need to clarify the situation with the relatives.

Should Clinicians Disagree?

Professional autonomy allows physiotherapists the freedom not to treat the patient in situations where it is assessed that treatment is inappropriate or contraindicated, despite the doctor's request.

- Discuss your concerns with the doctor.
- Why does the doctor feel that treatment is indicated?
- Could further investigations, such as chest X-ray, be performed to give clarity to the situation?

If you are still unhappy, you may wish to phone a senior physiotherapist for support and guidance.

When to Seek Help?

Remember that other members of the multidisciplinary team and your senior colleagues are there to support you. You must recognize the boundaries of your experience. In certain situations you should seek this support:

- If the patient is deteriorating rapidly. Following assessment you consider the patient is too unstable to tolerate any treatment and may require transfer to critical care for further medical management.

- Following assessment you are unable to identify the problem. Therefore you are uncertain about the correct management of the patient. Seek guidance from within the team.
- You are unsure as to specific modifications required to a planned treatment, for example the patient has recently undergone upper GI surgery and suction is indicated. Are there any precautions you should be aware of? If in doubt discuss the risk/benefits of the situation with a member of the medical team.
- To ascertain the patient's resuscitation status. If the patient is unstable there is a risk of respiratory or cardiac arrest during your treatment. Check in the nursing or medical notes. If you are unclear discuss with nursing staff or doctor. Make sure that this is the most recent decision.
- You have identified the problem but feel that the required treatment is outside your scope of practice. Call a colleague for support and advice. This must be discussed with the lead on call clinician the next day and a learning action plan agreed and implemented.

CONSENT

- We have a legal requirement to obtain consent to treat. Before you examine, treat or care for adult patients you must obtain their consent. Consent may be given in written, verbal or non-verbal form. This must be clearly documented in the patient's treatment record.
- The patient must be given a full explanation of the proposed treatment and any possible side-effects.
- Competent adult patients are entitled to refuse treatment, even when it would clearly benefit their health. The only exception to this is where the treatment is for a mental disorder and the patient is detained under the Mental Health Act 1983. This should be clearly documented in the patient's treatment records and discussed with the medical team.

Challenges to obtaining consent in the on call situation include:

Difficulty for the Patient Receiving Information
- hearing loss
- non English-speaking
- use of jargon.

Difficulty Interpreting Information
- depth of sedation
- cognitive impairment
- confusional state
- clinical depression.

Difficulty Responding to Information
- mechanical speech deficit (ET/trache tube)
- neurological speech deficit
- non English-speaking
- breathlessness/extreme fatigue.

Consider:

- How much time do you have to improve the quality of consent before the delay causes significant deterioration in the respiratory condition?
- Can any of the blocks to communication be removed or lessened within the time available before deterioration?
- How should you respond to explicit patient wishes already documented in the notes? (Some patients may have planned for situations when they cannot direct their own care.)

Remember:
Do not attempt to resolve complex issues of consent on your own. Always check your reasoning and judgement with the team in charge of the patient's care.

- Check your own organization's policy on consent and be aware of the CSP core standards and rules of professional conduct (January 2002). Advice is available on the Department of Health's website (www.doh.gov.uk/consent).
- Where it is not possible to gain consent, think about the following:
  a. Are you truly acting in the patient's best interests?
  b. Can you justify and document your reasons for giving or withholding care?
  c. Would your behaviour be acceptable to the majority of your professional peers?

DEALING WITH CHILDREN ON CALL

Staff are often more apprehensive about a call out to paediatric wards. During the on call situation there are some additional considerations (see also Chapter 3):

- You should attend mandatory child protection training. Different levels of training are required depending upon your level of involvement in paediatric care. Refer to your local policy.
- Discuss the child's home situation with the nursing staff. Who are the child's legal guardians? There may be a court order preventing the parents seeing the child. In this situation you must not discuss your treatment or the child's condition with the parents. Liaise only with the nursing staff or guardian *ad litem*.
- Children are likely to deteriorate much more rapidly than adults. You may have to assess and treat much more quickly.
- Depending on the age of the child, you may be unable to gain a subjective history. Use the parents or nursing staff to gain this information.
- The parents may help to reassure the child while you treat. Explain your role clearly and what your treatment involves. Ask if they would like to stay. Some parents may find treatment too distressing. In this situation a nurse who is familiar to the child will need to assist you.

ARRIVAL ON THE WARD

Organization

Following your arrival on the ward:

- Liaise with the nurse responsible for the patient's care.
- Review the medical notes.
- Review the physiotherapy notes.
- When was the patient last treated?
- What treatment modalities were used?
- Did the patient improve following the last physiotherapy intervention? How long was this improvement sustained?
- Identify the equipment you may need to treat the patient, e.g. oximeter, etc.

What to Do Next?

Having assessed, treated or not treated the patient, you should then:

- Discuss the outcome of your assessment and/or treatment with the nursing staff.

- Advise how nursing staff can maintain improvement (e.g. positioning, saline nebulizer, suction).
- Discuss when the patient will next receive treatment. Will you return later? Or under what circumstances should they call you again?
- Discuss with the patient or relatives when you will next treat.
- Leave a message for the day staff to identify that the patient should be seen early the following morning.
- Contact the switchboard to advise that you are leaving the site and return home to bed – hopefully to catch up on some much needed sleep!

ASSESSMENT

CHAPTER 2

Assessment of the adult patient

Hazel Horobin

This chapter considers the common presentation of the main respiratory problems, giving an overview of the essential areas of assessment and some common meanings of assessment findings. Normal values are given in bold text within square brackets (e.g. [37°C]). Further information can be found in Chapters 3, 4 and 5.

Remember:

- You are not alone in caring for this patient. You share the responsibility with the other members of the multidisciplinary team and can ask for help and information at any time.
- You will have begun the assessment during the telephone call. When you arrive on the ward, discuss the situation with the nurse looking after your patient. Before you look at the notes, glance at the patient. This will indicate how fast you need to act. If the patient seems very unwell, check:

  Airway: Are there any noises during respiration that indicate airway obstruction?

  Breathing: Is the patient breathing?

  Circulation: Is the CVS stable, does the patient look well perfused? (see Ch. 11.)

Ideally, you will have time to undertake a good 'paper' assessment of the patient using information from notes and charts. This will help guide your physical assessment.

COMMON PHYSIOTHERAPY PROBLEMS

Your assessment may highlight one or more of the problems listed in Table 2.1. Each usually presents in a specific pattern. Part of learning to assess cardiorespiratory patients is:

- recognizing these patterns
- developing a short list of options
- looking for evidence in the assessment to agree or disagree with them
- … leaving you with the most likely option/problem.

Table 2.1 Core problems: patterns of presentation

Symptom	Sputum retention (infection)	Volume loss	Pulmonary oedema	Broncho-spasm	Renal failure
↑ temperature – unless artificially lowered	Yes				
↑ WCC	Yes				
↓ PaO$_2$	Yes	Yes	Yes	Perhaps	
↑ PaCO$_2$ Hazard	If severe	If severe	If severe	If severe	
↓ PaCO$_2$	If ↑ RR			If ↑ RR	Yes = compensation
Acute ↑ HCO$_3^-$/H$^+$					Yes
Auscultation (see Ch. 4)	Crackles ↓ Breath sounds	↓ Breath sounds	Fine end inspiratory crackles	Wheeze	As pulmonary oedema if present
↓ Lung expansion	Perhaps	Yes			
Sputum colour	Yellow/green		White/pink		
Sputum consistency	Thicker		Frothy		
↑ WOB/↑ RR	Yes	Yes	Yes	Yes	Yes
CXR changes (see Ch. 5)	Perhaps	Yes	Yes	May be hyper-inflated	Yes if oedema
General medical history	?Respiratory disease ?Post-op. ?Smoke inhalation	?Post-op.	?Cardiac ?Renal	?Respiratory, e.g. asthma	?Renal

| Examples of recent occurrences | Pain, fear, immobility, dehydration, broncho-spasm, poor tidal volume/ cough, aspiration (see Ch. 6 for more detail) | Pain, fear, immobility (see Ch. 7 for more detail) | +ve fluid balance, ↑ JVP, poor urine output, recent i.v. fluids +, ↑weight | Infection, post-op., specific trigger | ↓ Urine output, acid base disturbance |

Remember:
- It is common for two or more problems to coexist.
- In each case you will see a combination of these patterns.
- The history will give you important clues as to the type of problem.
- Each patient will present slightly differently – look for the general trend.

THE CALL OUT

Consider:

- the reason for admission
- the reason for physiotherapy call out
- the subjective assessment
- the objective assessment – compared to the normal for that patient (Table 2.2).

Remember:
STOP
Look
Listen
Feel

Table 2.2 Assessment summary

Assessment	Potential assessment parameters
Database	Medical records, charts, monitors
Subjective	Current respiratory status, recent changes, usual status
Objective: Respiratory system	RR, observation, palpation, auscultation, CXR, level of oxygen received, oxygen saturation monitoring, arterial blood gases, assisted ventilation settings
Cardiovascular system	Heart rate, blood pressure, heart rhythm, bleeding from drains, other more complex monitoring, temperature, blood results – platelets, urea and creatinine
Neurological system	Consciousness, cooperation, intracranial pressure, cerebral perfusion pressure, Glasgow Coma Scale
Renal system	Urine output, fluid balance, renal function tests
Other	Other injuries Medication

Remember:

Highlight abnormal findings, contraindications and precautions. Then identify the key problems and the treatment plan.

MEDICAL RECORDS AND PATIENT CHARTS

Read the medical and physiotherapy notes (Table 2.3). For speed, read the initial admission notes, look for any summaries or major occurrences and read the current entry carefully.

Table 2.3 Information from notes

Information	Example content
History to date	• Reason for admission • Summary of events since admission • Speed and progression of deterioration • Normal physiological parameters for the patient
Significant past medical history	• Any concurrent pathology that affects the present situation (e.g. osteoporosis)
Drug history	• Usual medication • Newly prescribed drugs

Physiotherapy notes	• Previous problems identified • Treatments and outcomes? i.e. patient's tolerance • Is a similar treatment appropriate?
Other factors	• Resuscitation status • Psychosocial issues (e.g. patient awareness of diagnosis)

Patient's charts (Table 2.4) show:

• current physiological function
• trends over time.

Table 2.4 Information from patient's charts

Information	Relevance
Body temperature Core temperature **[37°C]**	>37.5°C = sign of infection – NB: note trends • Current temperature might be reduced as a result of therapy (e.g. paracetamol, fan application, CPAP, haemofiltration) rather than the absence of infection • Up to 1°C core temperature rise is normal within 24 h postoperatively • Potential sites of infection may be: a. chest b. wound c. urinary tract • Temperature increases metabolic demand and fluid loss • ↑WCC will confirm presence of infection **[4–11 × 10⁹ L]**
Cardiovascular system (CVS) Arterial blood pressure (BP) **[95/60–140/90 mmHg]**	Indicator of cardiovascular stability and function • Can anything account for sudden changes, e.g. positioning, drug change, line occlusion? • Does treatment benefit outweigh risk? • Treat people with a systolic BP of less than 90 mmHg or a diastolic BP of greater than 95 mmHg with care • Before beginning treatment discuss with nursing staff to establish whether BP can be stabilized prior to and during treatment

table continues

Information	Relevance
Mean arterial blood pressure **[65–100 mmHg]**	Range stated for individual patient is most important
Heart rate **[50–100 b.p.m.]** • Trend • Tachycardia >100 b.p.m. • Bradycardia <50 b.p.m. Heart rhythm (ECG)	Indicates cardiovascular function and physiological stress • Can anything account for sudden changes? • Indicative of sepsis/shock, inadequate analgesia, anxiety or respiratory distress • Indicative of specific cardiac problems, can occur during suction • See Chapter 4 for detail
Jugular venous pressure (JVP) or central venous pressure (CVP) **[3–15 cmH$_2$O]**	Indicates circulating blood volume • ↑ Suggests venous congestion secondary to fluid retention or heart failure • ↓ Suggests dehydration, a major bleed
Respiratory system (RS) Respiratory rate **[12–16 breaths/minute]**	**Causes of rapid respiratory rate = >20** • Respiratory problems • Anxiety/panic/pain • Metabolic problems Normal/near normal ABGs with a high respiratory rate can indicate an unsustainable degree of respiratory effort and impending respiratory failure **Causes of slow respiratory rate = <8** • Over-sedation • Neurological incident • Fatigue Discuss promptly with the medical team, particularly in the case of a rising PaCO$_2$
Oxygen saturation **[96–100%]**	• Blood oxygenation can give inaccurate readings if patient's circulation is peripherally shut down (indicated by cold hands and feet) or has a low haemoglobin level • Good monitoring device during treatment once reliability is established and acts as a good 'rough' guide to progression of respiratory problems and the outcome of treatment

	• Accept lower values (but not less than 80%) in chronic lung disease *depending upon the patient's normal saturations*
Arterial blood gases (ABGs): PaO₂ **[10.7–13.3 kPa (80–100 mmHg)]** PaCO₂ **[4.7–6.0 kPa (35–45 mmHg)]**	• See Chapter 4 for detailed analysis • Always view ABGs in relation to the oxygen being given (oxygen % or fraction of inspired oxygen – FiO₂) as an indicator of the severity of the problem, e.g. patient with low PaO₂ on high FiO₂ indicates a seriously ill person
pH [7.35–7.45]	pH below normal range requires immediate attention
Chest X-ray	See Chapter 5
Bronchoscopy or biopsy	There may be test results available – ensure patient is aware of result before discussing
Sputum culture	May require a specimen
Lung functions tests:	Important for long-term management. Only those listed below are important within the on call setting:
• Peak flow rates	Useful with asthmatics – indicates degree of bronchospasm and can be compared to normal
• Forced vital capacity (FVC)	Important with high spinal lesions or patients with Guillain–Barré syndrome (mechanical ventilation indicated if FVC is <1 L)
Respiratory system (ventilated patient) Mode of intubation: • Tracheostomy	May be less sedated and more able to cooperate with treatment
• ET tube (ETT) Mode of ventilation	Likely to be sedated – if not reassure + + • There are many types of ventilatory support. Discuss your individual patient's ventilatory needs with the nurse • See Chapter 9 • Poor patient/ventilator synchronization can result in respiratory distress and ineffective ventilation • May indicate what respiratory effort the patient can contribute

table continues

Information	Relevance
Peak airway pressures **[Alarm upper limit usually set at 40 mmHg]**	↑ May be due to: • Bronchospasm • Patient resistance • Sputum plug • Poor lung compliance, e.g. pulmonary oedema, fibrosis, ARDS ↑ Leads to: • ↑ Risk of pneumothorax • Long-term lung damage • Ineffective gas exchange due to poor perfusion
	Treat with care
Positive end expiratory pressure (PEEP)	If >10 cmH$_2$O: • Manual hyperinflation (MHI) not generally appropriate • Over 15 cmH$_2$O MHI is contraindicated
	Avoid disconnecting the patient from the ventilator if PEEP >10 cmH$_2$O
	• Closed suction systems will generally be used to maintain PEEP
FiO$_2$	Disconnect the patient from the ventilator with caution if on >0.6 FiO$_2$
Inspiratory:expiratory ratio **[Usually 1:2]**	Extended inspiratory time (e.g. 2:1 ratio) = attempt to improve gas diffusion in non-compliant lungs
	With inverse 2:1 ratio MHI is not appropriate
Central nervous system (CNS)	
Glasgow Coma Scale (GCS) **[3–15]**	Degree of awareness or responsiveness • Lower values indicate a less responsive patient
History of loss of consciousness?	• Head injury or brain surgery – see Chapter 13
Changing level of consciousness?	• Why? • Sedation related? • Deteriorating physiological condition?
Intracranial pressure (ICP) **[<10 mmHg, <1.3 kPa]**	See Chapters 4 and 13

Renal system	
Urine output **[1 ml/kg/h]**	↑ Or ↓ indicates fluid balance or renal problems: • Poor renal function will present with ↑ urea and creatinine levels Urea **[2.5–6.5 mmol/L]** Creatinine **[60–120 μmol/L]**
Overall fluid balance **[500–700 ml positive/24 h]**	Normally positive to account for difficult-to-measure daily losses (e.g. sweat) • >Fluid retention • <Dehydration See also Chapter 4
Blood results Platelets **[150–400 × 10⁹/L]** INR test **[1]** Haemoglobin (Hb)	**(Relevance within 24 h)** ↓ Platelets or ↑INR = potential problems with bleeding – a hazard for some treatments (check local policy) Leads to a reduced O₂ carrying capacity
Men **[14–18 g/100 ml]** Women **[11.5–15.5 g/100 ml]**	Visible symptoms: • Palor • Breathlessness
Urea **[2.5–6.5 mmol/L]** Creatinine **[60–120 μmol/L]**	↑ = Evidence of fluid balance or renal problems
Electrolytes: Potassium (K⁺) **[3.5–5.0 mmol/L]** Sodium (Na⁺) **[134–140 mmol/L]**	Abnormal levels in either direction have an impact on physiological (particularly cardiac) functioning

SUBJECTIVE ASSESSMENT

Detailed subjective examination is often not possible, but you should always:

• explain who you are and why you are there
• reassure the patient

before asking any questions (Table 2.5).

Table 2.5 Questions to consider asking

Questions	Response and possible indication
Are you in pain? Where, when, how bad? Does the pain allow cooperation with treatment? If not, more/alternative analgesia required?	Inspiratory pain, inadequate analgesia? • Wound pain • Fractured ribs • Pleural inflammation • Infection • Muscular Central sternal in absence of a sternal wound: • Cardiac pain?
Have you slept?	No: • Exhaustion? (Rest will be an important part of the plan if appropriate) Yes, but still sleepy: • Over analgesed • High CO_2
Can you move?	Pain and moving and handling risk assessment
Can you cough? Are you coughing anything up?	• Awareness of how to clear secretions and perception of ability • Look at sputum cleared for colour, viscosity
Are you drinking? (Only if patient allowed!)	Adequate hydration
If had previous physiotherapy: what works for you?	Some patients (e.g. CF patients) know their physiotherapy routine well

PHYSICAL ASSESSMENT

Comprises:

• observation (Table 2.6)
• palpation (Table 2.7)
• auscultation (Table 2.8).

Table 2.6 Observation

Details/environment	Concern
Oxygen	• Is FiO_2 maintaining adequate oxygenation? (All changes must be discussed with the doctor) • Adequate humidification? • Is the patient tolerating the mask or equivalent?

CPAP/non-invasive ventilation	• As above
	• Check settings – are they as prescribed?
	• How does the patient cope off the support (e.g. do saturations drop significantly)?
	NB Have extra O_2 available if you need to remove the device
Nasogastric tubes	• Probable reduced oral fluids
	• Make coughing and expectoration harder
Chest drains	See Chapter 14
Monitoring	Note pre-treatment levels to assess effect of treatment

The patient	Implication
Responsiveness	Level of consciousness and potential patient involvement in treatment influences treatment choices
Position	Does it facilitate resolution of the problem?
	• Hypoxaemia – V/Q matching principles
	• ↑WOB – ensure well supported position (p. 254)
	• Postural drainage appropriate to need
	• Loss of volume – positioning for best lung volume
	• Is the patient comfortable?
Chest movement:	
↑	• WOB
	• Anxiety
↓	• Low arousal
	• Pain
	• Atelectasis/volume loss
	• Chest wall trauma, deformity or disease
Unequal	• Unilateral pathology
Respiratory rate (RR)	• >30 breaths/min and increasing = **critical**
	• >40 breaths/min cannot be sustained
	• <8 risk of hypoventilation and CO_2 retention
Pattern of breathing	Pursed lip breathing and use of accessory muscles of respiration demonstrates ↑WOB:
	• Neck and arm muscles to aid inspiration
	• Abdominal contraction to aid expiration
Psychological distress	• Anxiety and fear
	• Restlessness
	• Claustrophobia, sometimes expressed as an intolerance of face masks and other O_2 equipment

table continues

The patient	Implication
Chest shape – any obvious chest/spinal deformity?	• Will ↑WOB • Causes a restriction of lung volume • A relatively minor infection may have a dramatic impact on patients whose respiratory load is always high
Gross nutritional status	• Will affect healing, energy, muscle strength

Cyanosis:
  Central
  Peripheral
	• Profound hypoxaemia
	• Can be an early sign of hypoxaemia, but more usually indicates poor peripheral circulation

Oedema:
  Legs (bilateral)
 	
  Total body
 	
  Just one limb
	• Right-sided cardiac failure, congestive cardiac failure, fluid overload or lack of muscle tone/leg movement
	• Frequently seen on ITU
	• Hypostatic oedema
	• Gross circulatory and/or fluid balance mechanism disturbance
	• Possible DVT, lymphoedema

Hands:
  Nails
  Tremor
 	
  Colour
	• Nail clubbing may indicate chronic problem
	• Twitch – narcotic flap sometimes seen in CO_2 retention
	• Fine – often a side-effect of bronchodilators
	• Nicotine stains indicate smoking history

Sputum:
  Colour
 	
  Volume
 	
  Consistency
	• Yellow/green = infection
	• White mucoid = chronic sputum overproduction
	• White frothy/watery = oedema or saliva
	• Pink frothy = severe pulmonary oedema
	• Blood streaks = inflammation of the airways
	• Significant amounts fresh blood = bleeding, pulmonary embolism or erosion of a pulmonary vessel
	• Grey = smoke inhalation/cigarettes/occupational history
	• How does volume expectorated relate to what you can hear on auscultation?
	• Very thick = poor humidification, infection or dehydration

Table 2.7 Palpation

Palpation	Rationale
Chest movement Is expansion adequate?	• Is it limited?
Is expansion equal?	• Unequal = unilateral problem or one side worse
	• Does this confirm what you observe?
Timing?	• Inspiratory:expiratory ratio **[1:2]**
Other palpable features of the chest wall	• Rate
	• Coordination of breathing
Is sputum palpable?	• Feels like a 'buzz' under your hands
Skin 'crackle'	• Surgical emphysema, air in the tissues = break in pleural continuity, can occur in trauma and around chest drains – not serious, but if gross is unpleasant and will reduce impact of positive pressure treatments
Any odd grating?	• Fractures, costal cartilage problems
	• Pleural inflamation
Temperature of extremities:	
Cold	• Peripheral circulation shut down
Very warm	• CO_2 retention, occasionally malignant hyperpyrexia (post acute head injury)
Skin quality	• If pinched skin remains creased = dehydration

Table 2.8 Auscultation

Auscultation	See Chapter 4 Listen for: • Breath sounds • Added sounds

PUTTING IT ALL TOGETHER

You now have much information from which to build a clinical picture and on which to base your treatment. This section helps you place your findings into symptom patterns common to the respiratory patient.

You have highlighted all abnormal/important information. Note which match with the patterns shown earlier (remember, you may be seeing a mixed picture – do not worry about this).

There are essentially only a few types of acute physical occurrences in the lungs:

Acute Physical Occurrences in the Lungs

Occlusive Material

Material can occlude the airways and airspaces, e.g.:
- infection (this may be mobile or consolidated):
  a. mucus in the airways
  b. inflammatory products in the alveoli
- blood
- material, e.g. tumour or an inhaled object (foreign body)
- oedema
- aspirated food/vomit, etc.

Changes in Volume

The volume of air they contain can alter, e.g.:
- Air in pleura may reduce lung volume.
- Chest wall movement may be limited because of:
  a. pain/surgery
  b. poor muscle function
  c. restricted chest movement.
- Lung may be consolidated (e.g. pneumonia).
- Lung may have collapsed.

Bronchospasm

Smooth muscle in the walls of the bronchial tree can spasm.

Problems Elsewhere in the Body

A problem elsewhere in the body (e.g. renal, cardiac) may be showing similar symptoms:
- renal
- cardiac
- acid–base compensation.

Further Reading

Hough A (2001) Physiotherapy in respiratory care, 3rd edn. Cheltenham: Stanley Thornes.

Pryor JA, Prasad SA (eds) (2002) Physiotherapy for respiratory and cardiac problems, 3rd edn. London: Churchill Livingstone.

Paediatric specifics

CHAPTER
3

Fiona Roberts

Although children develop the same respiratory problems as adults they are not miniature adults.

Age alters anatomy and physiology predisposing children to respiratory complications. Intervention must be adapted to accommodate these changes.

The differences are highlighted in this chapter.

CONSENT

- Consent is a legal requirement.
- Children under 16 years of age can give consent provided they fully understand what is involved.
- An adult with parental responsibility can give consent if the child is unable to do so.
- If an emergency arises and the child is unable to give consent and/or someone with parental responsibility is unavailable it is 'acceptable to undertake treatment to preserve life or prevent serious damage to health' (DoH 2001).
- Children sometimes refuse consent because they are frightened or do not understand.

COMMUNICATING WITH A CHILD

When assessing a child:

- Remember, the child may be very frightened, which can result in poor compliance.
- Use language appropriate to the child's stage of development.
- Persuasion may be necessary.
- Distraction and/or rewards may enhance compliance.
- Involving the child's parents may help; get them to demonstrate, coax, explain, etc.

PARENTS

- If they are present, parents will be very concerned, anxious and possibly frightened.
- These emotions can manifest themselves in many different ways.
- Always remember this if parents react in an unexpected way.
- Use tact and understanding with them.
- Always explain who you are and what you are going to do in a way that they will understand.

RESPONSE TO $\downarrow O_2$ (HYPOXAEMIA)

- Infants have higher metabolic oxygen consumption rates than adults.
- Hypoxia can, therefore, develop rapidly.
- The infant's response to hypoxia is to drop the heart rate to below 100 beats per minute (b.p.m.) (bradycardia).
- This can trigger pulmonary vasoconstriction which worsens the oxygenation status by limiting blood flow through the lungs.

ANATOMICAL AND PHYSIOLOGICAL DIFFERENCES IN CHILDREN

Anatomical and physiological differences resolve as children age but have significant influence on respiratory problems particularly in children under 5 years of age.

The first three differences listed in Table 3.1 prevent young children from increasing tidal volume (TV) as a means of increasing minute

Table 3.1 Effect and clinical implications of anatomical differences

Difference	Effect	Clinical implications
Ribs more horizontal in infants	No bucket handle effect	• Reduced ability to change thoracic cage diameter
Rib cage more compliant due to immature bone formation (rigidity increases as child reaches 8 years of age)	Less thoracic stability	• When respiratory load increases, pressure changes result in in-drawing of soft tissue (i.e. recession) • When positioning, dependent lung may be compressed and compromised

		• May make manual techniques more effective • Vibrations may cause atelectasis, as they reduce functional residual capacity (FRC)
Respiratory muscles contain fewer slow twitch fibres (adult 55%, child 30%)	Muscles will fatigue more quickly	• Very limited respiratory reserve • Respiratory fatigue develops very rapidly • Prompt and appropriate intervention required to prevent distress developing into fatigue
Intercostal muscles lack tone, power, coordination	Unable to provide significant assistance when respiratory load increases Do not help to provide thoracic stability	• Intercostal recession results
Heart:lung ratio relatively larger in infants (i.e. 1:1 compared to $\frac{1}{3}$:$\frac{2}{3}$ in adults)	Less space for lungs	• If heart size increases lungs will be compromised

volume (MV). To achieve this they increase respiratory rate while trying to maintain the same tidal volume. This increases respiratory muscle work and thus fatigue is likely.

Table 3.2 lists differences in the airways.

Remember:
Prone positioning provides thoracic stability and facilitates diaphragm function.

Hazard:
The possibility of sudden infant death syndrome means that babies should not be left prone without monitoring (e.g. apnoea alarm, pulse oximeter).

Table 3.2 Effect and clinical implications of airway differences

Airway differences	Effect	Clinical implications
Infants and babies have relatively larger tongues in comparison with adults	Predominantly nose breathers	• If nose is obstructed with secretions work of breathing can increase • Nasogastric tubes (NGTs) can have the same effect
Small airway diameter (infant trachea = 5–6 mm, adult trachea = 14–15 mm)	Increases resistance to airflow	• Small changes in airway diameter significantly increase resistance • Obstruction occurs more easily which will increase work of breathing, reduce lung volumes
Trachea's narrowest point: cricoid cartilage	Unable to use cuffed endotracheal tube (ETT) as this will cause damage	• Bypassing of secretions up sides of ETT • Also risk of vomit, and oral secretions, reaching lungs • Any trauma will lead to significant oedema and airway obstruction (see box below – stridor)
Floppy cartilage in trachea	Poor airway support	• Predisposed to airway collapse • Bronchodilators can worsen this – use with caution!
Immature cilia	Reduced efficiency of mucociliary transport	• Risk of infection • Reduced ability to cope with increased secretion quantity • Increased risk of retained secretions and airway collapse
Fewer, smaller alveoli (increase in numbers until 10–12 years then increase in size only)	Reduced gas exchange area	• Small amount of collapse/consolidation can cause significant changes in respiratory status (e.g. hypoxaemia, increased work of breathing)

Hazard:
Stridor (narrowing of upper trachea and/or larynx, usually heard on inspiration) can be caused by: trauma, infection, foreign body or congenital problems.

Do not treat unless origin is known and physiotherapy will not worsen condition.

Summary

To summarize these differences:

- More prone to atelectasis and retained secretions.
- Will fatigue quickly.
- Deterioration (and improvement) can be rapid.

OTHER DIFFERENCES

Older children usually demonstrate the same signs of respiratory distress as adults (Ch. 2).

Signs of respiratory distress seen in young children and babies are shown in Table 3.3.

Table 3.3 Signs of respiratory distress in young children and babies[a]

Signs of respiratory distress	Cause	Other information
Recession: a. intercostal b. subcostal c. sternal d. suprasternal (tracheal tug) e. supraclavicular	Identified areas sucked inwards during inspiratory pressure change due to lack of thoracic stability/muscle tone	• Mild/moderate/severe grades • Seen in babies, young children and those unable to fix their thoracic cage
See-sawing	Forceful contraction of diaphragm Causes abdomen to be pushed out and generates massive negative pressure in thorax sucking chest wall in	! Unsustainable • If observed immediate intervention required • Call medical staff
Nasal flare	Primitive response to entrain more air	• No actual effect

table continues

Signs of respiratory distress	Cause	Other information
Head bobbing	Attempt to use accessory respiratory muscles but unable to fix	• Sometimes seen as rotation if supine
Neck extension	Trying to reduce airflow resistance to reduce work of breathing	• In intubated children can be an attempt to get away from ETT • Could also be due to abnormal tone • Determine cause to enable appropriate intervention
Expiratory grunting	Trying to increase intrinsic positive end expiratory pressure (PEEP) and reduce work of breathing	• Increases FRC • Severe if audible at bedside • Less severe if only audible with stethoscope

a You may not see all of these signs together.

Handy Hint:
Babies/children with chronic respiratory problems may normally show some of these signs. It is important to compare their current signs with normal to identify if you should be concerned.

Cyanosis (blue discolouration to mucous membranes) is an unreliable sign of hypoxaemia in babies and infants due to the amount and type of haemoglobin in their blood.

Handy Hint:
There is no significant respiratory problem:
• if a child is sitting up/chatting/playing or if a baby is able to take a bottle.
Hazard:
If the child/infant is completely focused on breathing there is significant respiratory failure and prompt action is required.

ASSESSMENT

When assessing children we use all the information discussed in Chapter 2 and some specific to paediatrics. Some subjective information may be gained from the child, if you are able to ask the child directly, or from the parents/carer.

Additional subjective information from medical notes is listed in Table 3.4. Other subjective information specific to children is shown in Table 3.5.

Table 3.4 Additional subjective information from medical notes

Information required	Clinical relevance

Birth history:
  Was child born prematurely?
  Postnatal problems?
  Ventilation?
  Lung condition?
	• Preterm babies may have chronic lung conditions (e.g. bronchopulmonary dysplasia (BPD)) which cause poor lung compliance and impair gas exchange
	• May normally have: recession, long-term oxygen therapy (LTOT), secretions, raised CO_2, increased respiratory rate (RR)
	• BPD babies often do not tolerate handling
	• Respond with desaturation, bradycardia, apnoea
	• Prone to further respiratory problems mainly during first 12–18 months of life
	• Little respiratory reserve so fatigue rapidly
	• Need to be cautious using continuous positive airway pressure (CPAP) – risk of pneumothorax due to poor lung compliance

Any history of intraventricular haemorrhage or birth trauma?	• Can result in altered neurological status causing abnormal/delayed development
	• Abnormal development can result in:
	  a. poor cough
	  b. impaired swallow
	  c. poor airway protection
	• Can result in secretion problems and airway obstruction
	• May need to consider suction or tracheal rub

Pre-existing conditions?	• Significant chest or spinal deformities can alter lung mechanics • Some conditions result in respiratory muscle weakness (e.g. muscular dystrophy and spinal muscular atrophy)

table continues

Information required	Clinical relevance
	• Predisposes to respiratory complications and can also result in ineffective cough • Problems with positioning – may need to use support (e.g. pillows $++$)
Any history of gastro-oesophageal reflux (GOR)?	• If diagnosed, position with head up to prevent aspiration • Recurrent chest problems may be due to GOR

Table 3.5 Other subjective information specific to children

Information	Clinical relevance
Tolerance of handling: Does the child/infant desaturate? How quickly and to what level? Speed of recovery? Does the child/infant become bradycardic? Self-resolving or requiring stimulation to resolve? When was the child/infant last handled? Recovery time?	• Usually indicates: a. how sick the child is – commonly sicker children handle badly (e.g. desaturate, become bradycardic) b. degree of oxygen dependency • If handled recently and responded badly consider rest period before any intervention • Implications for how much assessment and/or treatment will be tolerated • Consider incorporating recovery time into assessment/treatment
Social history – including development	• If parents/carers present: who are you speaking to? • Do they have parental responsibility? • Consent? • Relevant information: e.g. care orders, psychological issues with child? • Influence approach to child • What can the child do for you?
Feeds: Bottle-feeding? Nasogastric tube feeding? Bolus or continuous? Feeds stopped?	• Inability to suck a bottle indicates shortness of breath (SOB) • Abdominal distension impairs diaphragm function • Continuous NG feeds/no feeds reduce diaphragmatic compromise • Those with severe respiratory distress will be on continuous or no feed

If on bolus feeds when was last one?	• Leave intervention for at least 1 h after feed to prevent vomiting

Signs of pain? Some children cannot express pain verbally. Look for other signs:
    Thumbs tucked in fist
    Frown
    Lethargy
    Irritability
	• Be observant and aware of the possible signs
	• Missing these signs will cause more pain if moving/treating child

OBJECTIVE INFORMATION

Factors with special significance in the assessment of children are shown in Table 3.6.

Table 3.6 Findings of special significance in the assessment of children

Objective finding	Change and clinical significance
Temperature	• Pyrexia can induce febrile convulsions in young children and babies • Child will be very sleepy after fitting • If pyrexial do not cover child/baby up or obstruct fan • Low temperature in a baby can increase oxygen requirements
CVS: heart rate and blood pressure Bradycardia	• Normal values alter with age (see Ch. 4) • Indicative of fatigue and/or hypoxaemia • If not self-resolving may require stimulation (pat on the bottom, rub chest) and increased supplemental oxygen
Respiratory rate: apnoeas – more than 20 seconds between breaths	• Values change with age (see Ch. 4) • Apnoeas can indicate respiratory distress, secretions or sepsis • May require stimulation (as for bradycardia)
Oxygen saturations	• Same as adult unless treating child with cyanotic cardiac defect (will have predetermined acceptable levels) (see Ch. 16)
Oxygen device adequate?	See Table 3.7

table continues

Objective finding	Change and clinical significance

Endotracheal tubes (ETT)	• Children nasally intubated unless contraindicated (e.g. skull fracture)
	• Provides greater security for ETT
	• Predisposed to:
	  a. airway leaks
	  b. bypass of secretions

Tracheostomy	• Unusual in children: once removed tracheostomy site can cause tracheal stenosis
	• If present means:
	  a. long-term airway problems
	  b. very long-term ventilation

Fluid balance	• Children are much smaller; therefore smaller positive volumes can be significant for them • Urine output usually 1–2 ml/kg/h • Positive volume of 200 ml significant for a small baby, insignificant for an 8 year old • Large positive balance – makes secretions very loose/causes pulmonary oedema • Negative balance – could cause tenacious secretions

OXYGEN DELIVERY

Table 3.7 Clinical implications of oxygen delivery devices

Device	Clinical implications
Masks	• Too big for babies • Babies/infants often dislike masks
Blow/flow by	• Mask placed near baby's face • Entrains large volume of air from environment with each breath, reduced oxygen content
Head box	• Plastic box with oxygen piped in. Placed over baby's head to provide an oxygen rich environment • Baby/infant may slide out towards opening for trunk • Oxygen concentration then lower due to ambient air entrainment
Nasal prongs	• Can be used even on babies. Direct administration to airway but limited flow possible

AUSCULTATION

There are several issues to consider when using auscultation on a child (Table 3.8).

Table 3.8 Issues to consider when using auscultation

Issue	Clinical implication
Secretions pool in posterior lung areas, especially bases, due to prolonged periods in supine position	• Must listen to posterior aspect of thorax
Small distance between upper airways and lungs	• Transmitted sounds common • Can be misleading • Always listen without stethoscope first then compare sounds
Adult stethoscopes cover large areas of thorax	• Difficult to localize problem area
Upper lobe common site of collapse/consolidation	• Listen to upper lobes anteriorly and posteriorly

COMMON CONDITIONS

Table 3.9 lists conditions commonly referred for on call physiotherapy and the implications they have for assessment.

Table 3.9 Common conditions referred for on call physiotherapy and their implications for assessment

Condition	Implications for physiotherapy
Bronchiolitis	• Physiotherapy not usually effective in acute phase • If ventilated, assess carefully. If area of reduced air entry and/or crackles on auscultation treat as appropriate as indicative of collapse and/or retained secretions • Whether ventilated or not, these babies often desaturate with handling
Whooping cough (pertussis)	• Physiotherapy contraindicated in acute stages • If ventilated, paralysed and sedated – treat if crackles indicating retained secretions or

table continues

Condition	Implications for physiotherapy
	reduced air entry indicating focal collapse found on assessment
Croup (acute laryngotracheobronchitis)	• Physiotherapy contraindicated in the non-intubated child
Acute epiglottitis	• Physiotherapy contraindicated in the non-intubated child • Only treat the intubated child if assessment indicates need
Pneumonia	• Active treatment only effective if assessment indicates sputum retention (crackles on auscultation)
Inhaled foreign body	• Only treat, if indicated, once foreign body has been removed by bronchoscope
Non-accidental injury (NAI)	• If child admitted with concerns of NAI be aware of neurological complications, e.g. signs of fitting, Glasgow Coma Score • May have rib fractures

Key messages

- Children are prone to atelectasis and retained secretions.
- Small areas of atelectasis or small amounts of secretions can cause significant deterioration in work of breathing and gas exchange.
- Children have poor respiratory reserves.
- If signs of respiratory distress (see below), intervene quickly.
- Bradycardia = hypoxia.
- If child is playing, chatting, taking a bottle with no problems there is no significant respiratory problem.
- Adapt your approach to suit the child's development.
- Keep parents informed.

Signs of Respiratory Distress in Children:

Recession

See-sawing

Nasal flare

Head bobbing
Neck extension
Expiratory grunting
Focused only on breathing.

References

Department of Health (2001) Seeking consent: working with children. DoH November 2001. http://www.doh.gov.uk/consent (consulted 28 June 2002).

Further reading

Aloan CA, Hill TV (1997) Respiratory care of the newborn and child, 2nd edn. Philadelphia: Lippincott, p. 97.

Assessment tools

Sandy Thomas

This chapter gives the normal values for clinical observations and tests (shown in square brackets in bold type), together with some suggestions about implications and interpretation. Abbreviations have been used in the tables where appropriate (please see the list of abbreviations in Appendix 3, p. 301).

The chapter deals with the following topics:

- auscultation
- oximetry
- arterial blood gases and other blood measurements
- respiratory monitoring
- neurological monitoring
- cardiovascular monitoring
- electrocardiograms (ECGs).

AUSCULTATION (Table 4.1)

A good technique is important. Ensure that you make time to practise this in your induction and at regular updates.

Table 4.1 Notes on auscultation

Auscultation	
Normal breath sounds	• Soft, muffled • Louder in inspiration, fade in expiration • Ratio 1:2
Bronchial breathing: • Louder, coarse, on expiration and inspiration, with pause between • Heard normally over trachea	If heard over lung fields, suggests: • Consolidation and/or • Collapse *(Providing airway not completely blocked)* • At fluid line of pleural effusion

Breath sounds quiet or absent?	**Possible causes:** • Shallow breathing • Poor positioning • Atelectasis/collapse • Collapse with complete obstruction of airway • Sounds filtered by air (hyperinflation) • Sounds filtered by pleura, chest wall (obese or muscular patients, pleural effusion, pneumothorax, haemothorax)
Absent breath sounds *with* hyper-resonant percussion note	**Hazard:** Pneumothorax
Crackles	Short, non-musical, popping sounds
During inspiration? Early inspiratory crackles	Reopening of larger airways
Late inspiratory crackles	Reopening of small, peripheral airways and alveoli **Possible causes:** • Low lung volumes • Atelectasis • Pneumonia • Pulmonary oedema • Fibrosis of lung parenchyma
During expiration?	May be sputum if: • Coarse sounding • Also in mid-inspiration • Change following coughing
Early in expiration	Sputum in central airways
Late in expiration	Sputum in more peripheral airways
Hint: Absence of expiratory crackles does not necessarily mean absence of secretions, as crackles are only heard if velocity of airflow is adequate and breath sounds audible	
Wheezes	Musical sounds due to vibration of wall of narrowed or compressed airway **Possible causes:** • Bronchospasm • Airway oedema • Sputum

table continues

Auscultation	
	• Tumour • Foreign body
Pleural rub Crackling or grating Identical in inspiration and expiration	• Inflammation of pleura
Percussion note	
Hollow sound and feel (resonant) due to air in thorax	• Air in lung (normal) Increased (hyper-resonant) in: • Emphysema (bullae) • Air between the pleura (pneumothorax)
A dull sound and flat feel due to fluid or solid	• Normal over liver or abdominal contents • Pleural effusion • Consolidation

OXIMETRY (Table 4.2)

Table 4.2 Notes on oximetry

SpO$_2$	[Normal range 95–98%]
• SpO$_2$ less than 90%	Significant hypoxaemia *but* see following
• Elderly patients and during sleep	Expect lower values
• Hb	Consider before interpreting SpO$_2$ as affects oxygen content
• Oxygen% *or* FiO$_2$ (ventilated patient)	Take into account any oxygen patient is receiving when interpreting SaO$_2$/PaO$_2$ Does oxygen therapy require medical review?
• Acute illness (acute asthma, pneumonia, infection, postop. atelectasis)	Below 92% may be significant in adults
• Chronic chest patient	Hypoxaemia may not be significant in adults until below 80–85%; compare with usual values for patient

ARTERIAL BLOOD GASES (AND BLOOD MEASUREMENTS) (Tables 4.3 and 4.4)

Critical gas levels are shown in Table 4.4. Note that paediatric values may differ (see Table 4.3 for ranges).

Table 4.3 Notes on arterial blood gases and blood measurements

Normal ranges		Implications
PaO_2		Low oxygen levels in blood = hypoxaemia
Adults	**[10.7–13.3 kPa (80–100 mmHg)]**	Significance depends on age and type of pathology (acute or chronic) – see below
Newborns	**[8–11 kPa (60–90 mmHg)]**	
Preterm babies	**[7–10 kPa (52–75 mmHg)]**	Note oxygen delivery
Infants 1–3 years	**[9–12 kPa (67–90 mmHg)]**	
Children over 3 years	**[12–14 kPa (90–105 mmHg)]**	
$PaCO_2$		
Adults and children over 3 years	**[4.7–6.0 kPa (35–45 mmHg)]**	
	• <4.7 kPa (35 mmHg) =	Hypocapnia (hyperventilation)
	• >6.0 kPa (60 mmHg) =	Hypercapnia (hypoventilation)
Babies and children under 3 years	**[4–4.7 kPa (30–35 mmHg)]**	
	• <4 kPa (30 mmHg) =	Hypocapnia (hyperventilation)
	• >4.7 kPa (35 mmHg) =	Hypercapnia (hypoventilation)
$PaCO_2$ levels in response to oxygen therapy in chronic chest patients	**Hazard:** If hypoxaemic and O_2 is increased check ABGs – that CO_2 has not climbed. Some patients with chronic respiratory disease may rely on their hypoxic drive to breathe; thus too much oxygen removes the drive to breathe (see Ch. 12)	

Table 4.4   Notes on critical gas levels[a]

Critical gas levels	
Acute patients (adults)	• Hypoxaemia <10.7 kPa (80 mmHg) is **significant** • Hypoxaemia <7.3 kPa (55 mmHg) **critical** • Hypercapnia – any measurement outside normal range is **significant**
Chronic patients (adults)	Critical levels depend on degree of compensation so compare with patient's usual values and their pH • Hypoxaemia <7.3 kPa (55 mmHg) **significant** • Hypercapnia >6.0 kPa (45 mmHg) **significant** if pH falls • Hypercapnia >8.0 kPa (60 mmHg) **critical** if pH falls

[a]Paediatric values may differ – see Table 4.3 for ranges.

Direction of Change in ABG Measurements in Acidosis and Alkalosis from Respiratory or Metabolic Causes
(Tables 4.5 and 4.6)

This categorization assumes that any compensation is complete, not partial:

• If compensation is only partial, pH is not completely restored to normal.
• Note that it may be impossible to distinguish between compensated respiratory acidosis and compensated metabolic alkalosis, or between compensated respiratory alkalosis and compensated metabolic acidosis, without looking at other clinical findings.

Table 4.5   Levels in acidosis and alkalosis

Description	pH	PaCO$_2$	HCO$_3^-$
Respiratory acidosis	Low	High	Normal
Respiratory alkalosis	High	Low	Normal
Metabolic acidosis	Low	Normal	Low
Metabolic alkalosis	High	Normal	High
Compensated respiratory acidosis	Normal[a]	High	High
Compensated respiratory alkalosis	Normal[a]	Low	Low
Compensated metabolic acidosis	Normal[a]	Low	Low
Compensated metabolic alkalosis	Normal[a]	High	High

[a]See Table 4.6.

Table 4.6   Normal ranges and implications

Normal ranges		Implications
pH (adults and children over 3 years	**[7.35–7.45]**	• Acidosis (<7.35) – **critical** may cause lethargy, disorientation or confusion, loss of consciousness • Alkalosis (>7.45) may lead to increased muscle tone and spasms • With abnormal pH, also check $PaCO_2$ and HCO_3^- to identify cause (respiratory or metabolic)
pH (babies and children below 3 years)	**[7.3–7.4]**	
HCO_3^- BE	**[22–26 mmol/L]** **[−2–+2]**	• High values (above 26 mmol/L or above +2 BE) suggest bicarbonate (base) has been retained. Makes blood more alkaline and raises pH (metabolic alkalosis) • Low values (below 22 mmol/L or below −2 BE) suggest bicarbonate (base) has been excreted. Makes blood more acidic and lowers pH (metabolic acidosis) • This is a longer acting compensatory mechanism
Hb	**[14–18 g/100 ml (men)]** **[11.5–15.5 g/100 ml (women)]** **[16–19 g/100 ml (newborns)]** **[13–15 g/100 ml (children)]**	• Low values (below 12.0 g/100 ml in adults) = anaemia, lowers oxygen carrying capacity. Consider haemoglobin levels when interpreting SaO_2 • High values (above 16.5 g/100 ml in adults) = polycythaemia, compensatory in chronic chest patients

Hint:
Cyanosis may not be evident in patients with low Hb, even with very low SaO_2 (although these patients may have critically low oxygen content), whereas patients with high levels of Hb may show cyanosis easily, but not be significantly hypoxaemic.

table continues

Normal ranges		Implications
Na$^+$	**[134–140 mmol/L]**	Hypernatraemia (>140 mmol/L): • Dehydration • Affects sputum clearance and patient stability Hyponatraemia (<134 mmol/L): • Overhydration • Pulmonary oedema
K$^+$	**[3.4–5.0 mmol/L]**	• Hypokalaemia (<3.4 mmol/L) • Hyperkalaemia (>5 mmol/L) Both cause cardiac instability due to dysrhythmias
Platelets	**[150–400 × 10^{-9}/L]**	Check your local policy as each unit may differ. The rule of thumb is <50 × 10^{-9}/L take extreme care and discuss all activities which may cause barotrauma (e.g. IPPB, suction, etc.) or bruising with the medical team – they will need to weigh up the risk/benefit to the patient. Treatment may be possible during platelet infusion (see Ch. 16 for more detailed advice)
WCC	**[4–11 × 10^{-9}/L]**	Above 11 × 10^{-9}/L indicates infection (chest/wound/urinary infection?)

RESPIRATORY MONITORING (Tables 4.7 and 4.8)

Table 4.7 Normal values and implications

Normal values		Implications
Respiratory rate: Adults Newborns Infants <6 years Children >6 years	 **[12–16]** **[30–50]** **[20–30]** **[15–20]**	• These are *resting* rates so expect increases when demand increases • Always relate to ABGs and other symptoms
Increased rate		• Hyperventilating? Check for low PaCO$_2$ (stress, anxiety, pain)

	• Increased demand? (Exercise, fever, increased work of breathing) • Less efficient ventilation (due to ↓tidal volume) at higher respiratory rates – fatigue likely • Low PaO_2 *and* high respiratory rate indicates cardiac or respiratory problem
>30 per min (in adults), trend *increasing*	Becoming **critical:** • Check gases and any signs of respiratory failure
Reduced rate RR <1 and trend *reducing*	Could be **critical:** • Over sedation? • Neurological incident? • Fatigue? • Check gases and look for any signs of respiratory failure

Table 4.8 Lung function tests

Lung function tests:
Vary with age, sex and height – *need to compare with predicted normals.* Values often found in notes as *percentage* of those predicted for patient's age, sex and height. Paediatric values differ and are not given here, but observe trends as these are more relevant in critical care than absolute values.

FVC	**[4–5 L (average adult male)]**	Values below 1 L may be critical and require ventilation in patients with muscle weakness and neurological conditions
FEV_1	**[Normally >70% of FVC]**	• <80% predicted airways obstruction (e.g. COPD) • 60–80% predicted = mild obstruction • 40–60% predicted = moderate obstruction • <40% predicted = severe obstruction
PEFR	**[5–8 L/s or 300–500 L/min]**	• <80% predicted suggests airways obstruction • Useful indication of severity of respiratory disease • Observe trend carefully in asthmatics as may deteriorate fast • Use bronchodilator before treatment if low

NEUROLOGICAL MONITORING

(Table 4.9; see also Ch. 14)

Table 4.9 Normal values and implications

Normal values		Implications
Glasgow Coma Scale (GCS)	**[Range 3–15 (adults and older children)]**	• <15 suggests *some* loss of conscious awareness • The lower the score, the less the response (minimum score is 3) • Consider trend for patient's prognosis
Intracranial pressure (ICP)	**[10 mmHg (1.3 kPa)]**	• >20 mmHg (2.7 kPa) **critical,** however, significance of increase depends on arterial blood pressure (and therefore CPP)
	Increased by	• Suction, change of position, tipped (head down) position, increased pain, neck rotation, poor MHI technique resulting in ↑CO_2, inadequate sedation – all may increase pressure in the cerebral vessels
	Decreased by	• Medication • Ventilation to hyperventilate (aim ↓CO_2) • See Chapter 14
Cerebral perfusion pressure (CPP) = MAP − ICP	**[>70 mmHg]**	• <50 mmHg **critical** • Suggests inadequate blood flow to the brain and likely neuronal damage • Check with team for agreed acceptable levels on your unit • May contraindicate most physiotherapy treatments

CARDIOVASCULAR MONITORING

(Table 4.10)

Table 4.10 Normal values and implications[a]

Normal values (ranges)		Implications
HR		
Preterm babies	[100–200 b.p.m.]	• Bradycardia <100 Tachycardia >200
Newborns	[80–200 b.p.m.]	• Bradycardia <80 Tachycardia >200
Infants <2 years	[100–190 b.p.m.]	• Bradycardia <100 Tachycardia >190

Infants
  >2 years
	[60–140 b.p.m.]	• Bradycardia <60
		  Tachycardia >140

Children
  2–6 years
	[60–90 b.p.m.]	• Bradycardia <60
		  Tachycardia >90

Adults	[50–100 b.p.m.]	• Bradycardia <50
		  Tachycardia >100
		  (See also section on ECG monitoring)

BP		• Increases with age; for systolic
Preterm babies	[39–59/ 16–36 mmHg]	values add person's age to 100 to estimate
Newborns	[50–70/ 25–45 mmHg]	• Significance of abnormal values depends on patient's normal.
Infants <2 years	[87–105/ 53–66 mmHg]	Note changes or trends
Infants >2 years	[95–105/ 53–66 mmHg]	
Children 2–6 years	[97–112/ 57–71 mmHg]	
Adults	[95–140/ 60–90 mmHg]	
	Hypotension	• <95/60 (adults) suggest onset of circulatory shock (**critical**) • Care with, or avoid physiotherapy until pressure stable
	Hypertension	• >140/90 (adults) may indicate hypertension although significance depends on patient's age and their usual values • >95 mmHg diastolic – treat with care
Mean arterial pressure (MAP) (adults)	[65–100 mmHg]	

table continues

Normal values (ranges)		Implications
Central venous pressure (CVP)	**[1–6 mmHg]** **[3–15 cmH₂O]** **Low values** <3 cmH₂O (1 mmHg) **High values** >15 cmH₂O (6 mmHg)	Indicates circulating blood volume • Suggest poor venous return • May be dehydrated • Suggest overhydration, cardiac failure (possible pulmonary oedema if left side of heart failing – check PAWP)
Pulmonary artery wedge pressure (PAWP)	**[5–12 mmHg (1.3–2.7 kPa)]**	If >12 mmHg (2.7 kPa) suggests: • Left-sided heart failure • Pulmonary oedema • Adult respiratory distress syndrome
Urine output	**[1 ml/kg/h]**	If <400 ml per day: • Renal failure, or • Fluid conservation due to dehydration or circulatory shock (check BP)
Fluid balance	**[Intake and output should roughly balance]** Input > output over 2–3 days suggests Output > input over a few days suggests	• Need to look at this over a couple of days • Patients also lose fluid via insensible fluid loss (e.g. sweat) each day • Fluid overload due to renal failure or heart failure • Possible pulmonary or peripheral oedema • Fluid depletion and dehydration • Dry viscous secretions • Possible hypovolaemic shock

ᵃEach patient may have individual ranges.

ECG MONITORING

(Figs 4.1–4.8)

- You are not responsible for diagnosis – ask for help if unsure.
- Look to see if trace is regular or not, and if it is fast or slow (Fig. 4.1).
- Patients respond differently to dysrhythmias and a serious dysrhythmia in one person may have no adverse effects in another, so look at patient and discuss with medical/nursing staff!

- Blood pressure is *the key* when deciding the importance of any dysrhythmia. Also consider general observations such as colour, temperature and consciousness level.
- The *trend* of any dysrhythmia is also important:
  a. has it just occurred?
  b. did it occur suddenly or gradually?
  c. is it getting more frequent?
  d. how is your treatment affecting it?
  e. pay attention to dysrhythmias which have recently appeared, or are getting more frequent.
- Manual chest treatments may affect the ECG tracing, so allow time for the tracing to settle before interpreting any abnormality.

Sinus Rhythm (Fig. 4.1) Normal tracing
Regular rate and pattern
between 60 and 100 beats
per minute

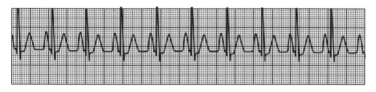

II

Figure 4.1 Rhythm strip to show sinus rhythm.

Possibly Serious Dysrhythmias
The following dysrhythmias may be unimportant for some patients, but may become **critical** in others:

Remember:
- Always consider patient's symptoms and blood pressure.
- If in doubt, ask another member of the team before treating.

Sinus Bradycardia (Fig. 4.2)
HR <50 beats per minute

- May be normal for some, e.g. those on betablocker medication
- Consider blood pressure
- Very low bradycardias may cause shock, but a low heart rate with a normal blood pressure is not cause for alarm

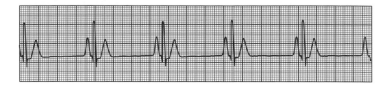

II

Figure 4.2 Rhythm strip to show sinus bradycardia.

	• Can occur during suction; preoxygenate patients to minimize the risk of a vasovagal response
Sinus Tachycardia (Fig. 4.3) HR >100 beats per minute	• Fever, pyrexia • Recent trauma or surgery • Pain, fear and anxiety • May cause no problems, but over 130/min affects efficiency of heart and may be dangerous for patients with cardiac disease • Consider predicted 'maximum' (220 − age) and decide how much leeway you have should physiotherapy further increase rate

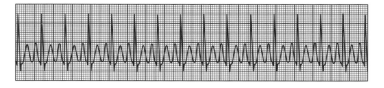

II

Figure 4.3 Rhythm strip to show sinus tachycardia.

Atrial Fibrillation (Fig. 4.4) Frequent irregular P waves appear as an erratic baseline	• Could be asymptomatic • May compromise BP, and thus • Could lead to problems with cardiac output during activity or increased demand • Increased risk of thrombus or embolus formation

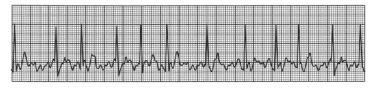

ll

Figure 4.4 Rhythm strip to show atrial fibrillation.

Ventricular Ectopics or Premature Ventricular Contractions (PVCs) (Fig. 4.5)
Irregular QRS complexes
May be premature, wider than usual and have a bizarre shape

May become **critical** if:

- Can occur in normals without adverse effects BUT
- May warn of severe dysrhythmias in patients with cardiac disease

- Increase in frequency (more than 6 per minute)
- Shape of each ectopic differs
- Several ectopics occur together in a row
- Increased frequency of ectopics can lead to ventricular tachycardia or ventricular fibrillation

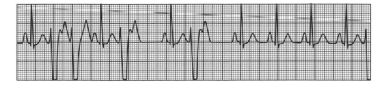

ll

Figure 4.5 Rhythm strip to show ventricular ectopics.

Serious Dysrhythmia

Warning:
The following dysrhythmia is usually serious – *always seek advice before treating.*

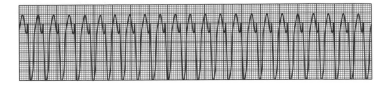

II

Figure 4.6 Rhythm strip to show ventricular tachycardia.

Ventricular Tachycardia (Fig. 4.6) Regular, fast (over 140 per minute) QRS complexes, without associated P wave	• Ectopic focus in ventricles • Serious dysrhythmia; may lead to ventricular fibrillation • Reduced cardiac output; may quickly become **critical**

Critical ECGs with No Cardiac Output

Hazard:

If you are the first on the scene and the patient is unresponsive, activate the buzzer/crash button immediately and start cardiopulmonary resuscitation (CPR).

Ventricular Fibrillation (VF) (Fig. 4.7) Unorganized, chaotic, irregular waves suggest that the ventricles are fibrillating	No cardiac output – patient will die within minutes unless rhythm is reversed by defibrillation

Asystole (flat line) (Fig. 4.8) Compete lack of electrical activity	No cardiac output – patient will die unless electrical activity can be restored *NB Check ECG leads as this can occur if they have become disconnected*

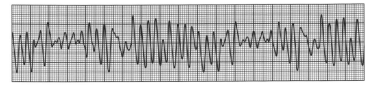

II

Figure 4.7 Rhythm strip to show ventricular fibrillation.

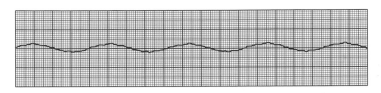

II

Figure 4.8 Rhythm strip to show asystole.

Further reading

Buchanon G, Smith M (1998) Electrocardiography. In: Smith M, Ball V (eds) Cardiovascular/respiratory physiotherapy. London: Mosby International, ch. 4.

Hough A (2001) Physiotherapy in respiratory care, 3rd edn. Cheltenham: Stanley Thornes.

Pryor JA, Prasad SA (eds) (2002) Physiotherapy for respiratory and cardiac problems, 3rd edn. London: Churchill Livingstone.

Wilkins RL, Jones Krider S, Sheldon RL (1995) Clinical assessment in respiratory care, 3rd edn. London: Mosby International.

CHAPTER 5 Chest X-ray interpretation

Stephen Harden

The emphasis of this chapter is the X-ray appearance of common conditions that you will see when on call. As the majority of patients requiring emergency physiotherapy are short of breath or have suboptimal gas exchange, only abnormalities of the lungs and pleural spaces are demonstrated. Only frontal X-rays (posteroanterior (PA) and anteroposterior (AP)) are used as these are the ones that you will be required to interpret.

Remember that a perfect chest X-ray (CXR; Fig. 5.1) requires correct patient positioning and the correct X-ray dose. Deficiency in any of

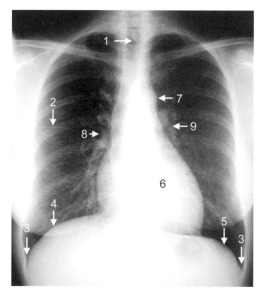

Figure 5.1 Normal chest X-ray.
Key: 1 trachea; 2 horizontal fissure; 3 costophrenic angle; 4 right hemidiaphragm; 5 left hemidiaphragm; 6 heart shadow; 7 aortic arch; 8 right hilum; 9 left hilum.

these results in a suboptimal X-ray and may produce appearances that simulate lung pathology.

NORMAL LOBAR ANATOMY

- The right lung contains three lobes, upper (RUL), middle (RML) and lower (RLL) (Fig. 5.2A–B).
- On the right side, the oblique fissure separates the RUL from the RLL above the horizontal fissure and the RML from the RLL below it.
- The horizontal fissure separates the RUL from the RML.

Remember:
When looking at a frontal CXR:
- RUL is at the top above the horizontal fissure
- RML is at the base anteriorly below the horizontal fissure
- RLL is posterior.

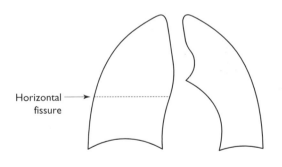

Figure 5.2A
Frontal plane.

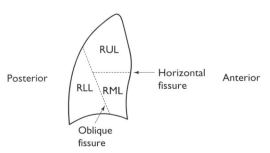

Figure 5.2B
Right lung, lateral.

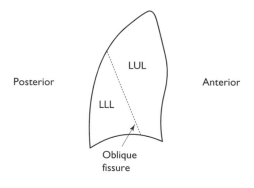

Figure 5.2C   Left lung, lateral.

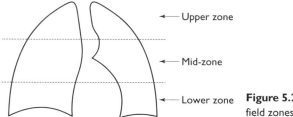

Figure 5.2D   Lung field zones.

- The left lung consists of two lobes, upper (LUL) and lower (LLL) (Fig. 5.2C). The lingula is the most inferior part of the LUL.
- The oblique fissure on the left side separates the LUL and LLL.

Remember:
The LUL is anterior and the LLL is posterior.

For descriptive purposes, the lungs on the CXR are divided into thirds or zones (Fig. 5.2D):

- upper zone
- mid-zone
- lower zone.

These are NOT ANATOMICAL divisions. For example, the apex of the lower lobe on each side is in the mid-zone.

HOW TO INTERPRET ABNORMALITIES IN THE LUNG FIELDS ON THE CXR

Essentially, these areas are abnormal because they appear either:
- too white

or
- too black.

Too White

The vast majority of abnormalities in the on call setting are areas that are too white and the commonest causes are:

- collapse or atelectasis
- consolidation
- pleural effusion
- pulmonary oedema.

Too Black

When there are areas which appear too black, the most important causes are:

- pneumothorax
- COPD.

Each of these is described below.

ATELECTASIS/COLLAPSE

Atelectasis or collapse refers to an area of lung which is airless and the lung collapses in this region. Atelectasis may involve an entire lobe or even an entire lung.

The chest X-ray will show a loss of lung volume. This means that the lung field will be smaller than expected. Other structures may move to fill up the space, so there may be:

- shift of the mediastinal structures such as the heart or trachea
- elevation of the hemidiaphragm compared to the other side.

The area of collapsed lung appears as a white or 'dense' area and this represents airless lung tissue. When this affects a small volume of the lung, the appearance is of a white line and this is often seen at the lung bases in postoperative patients. When a whole lobe collapses, each produces a specific appearance (Table 5.1):

Table 5.1 Appearance of lobe collapse

Lobe collapse	Presentation
RUL collapse	• There is increased density high in the right lung down to the horizontal fissure • This fissure swings upwards and can adopt an almost vertical position (Fig. 5.3)
RML collapse	• The RML collapses down against the right heart border which becomes indistinct (Fig. 5.4) • The right heart border is clearly seen on a normal CXR because it lies adjacent to the air-filled middle lobe
RLL collapse	• There is a triangular density low in the right lung but the right heart border can still be clearly seen (Fig. 5.5)
LUL collapse	• The left lung is slightly whiter than the right • The LUL is anterior and so collapses against the anterior chest wall. Thus, you see air in the LLL through the dense collapsed LUL (Fig. 5.6)
LLL collapse	• A triangular density is seen behind the heart (Fig. 5.7) • The part of the heart shadow to the left of the spine is whiter than that to the right of the spine

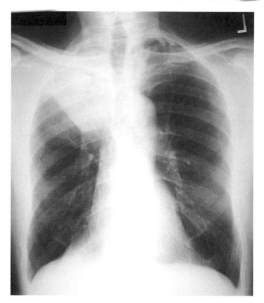

Figure 5.3 Right upper lobe collapse. The horizontal fissure is now orientated obliquely. The trachea is deviated to the right which is evidence of mediastinal shift.

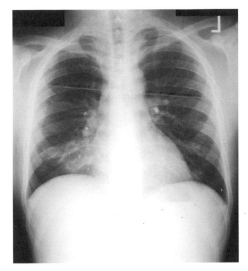

Figure 5.4 Right middle lobe collapse. The right heart border is indistinct and there is a vague white appearance to the adjacent lung.

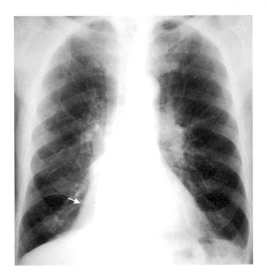

Figure 5.5 Right lower lobe collapse. There is abnormal whiteness with a straight outer border (arrow) low in the right lung. The right heart border is still visible.

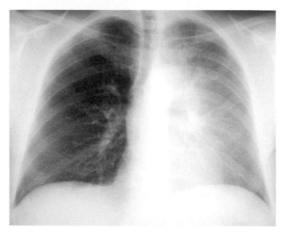

Figure 5.6 Left upper lobe collapse. There is a hazy increased whiteness over the left hemithorax. The left heart border is indistinct.

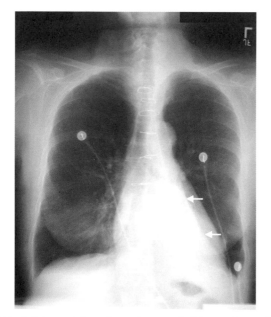

Figure 5.7 Left lower lobe collapse. Increased whiteness is seen behind the heart with a straight outer edge (arrows).

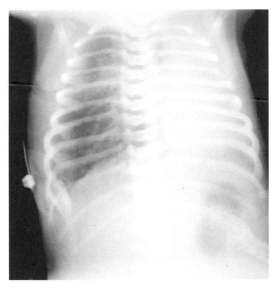

Figure 5.8 Left lung collapse. There is abnormal whiteness over the left hemithorax. The heart is shifted to the left within the abnormal area.

When a whole lung collapses there is increased density of the entire hemithorax (Figs 5.8 and 5.9). This appearance is sometimes called a 'white-out', although there are other causes for this. A pneumonectomy is in effect an extreme form of complete lung collapse and so will look the same on CXR but you may see rib irregularity marking the site of the thoracotomy.

Remember:
When you see complete collapse of the left lung associated with RUL collapse in a ventilated patient always check the position of the endotracheal tube. If the tube has been advanced down the right main bronchus then only the RML and RLL will be aerated (Fig. 5.10).

CONSOLIDATION

Consolidation occurs when air in lung is replaced by fluid. The distribution of this consolidation may be patchy or may affect an entire

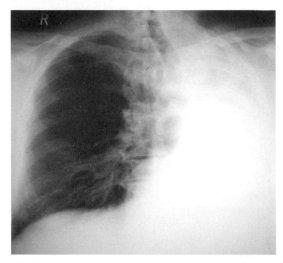

Figure 5.9 Pneumonectomy. Abnormal whiteness is seen in the left hemithorax. The trachea and heart are shifted to the left.

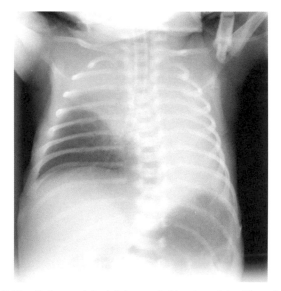

Figure 5.10 Collapse of the left lung and right upper lobe. Note the tip of the ET tube which lies in the right interlobar bronchus.

segment or lobe. The composition of this fluid depends on the cause:

- infected fluid, as in pneumonia (the commonest cause that you will see)
- saliva or gastric contents, seen in cases of aspiration
- blood, in cases of traumatic lung contusion
- serous transudate, seen in alveolar pulmonary oedema.

Although the distribution may help to elicit the cause, the radiological appearance of consolidation is the same for all of these:

Radiological Appearance
- The **whiteness or shadowing** in the lung is **poorly defined**. It is difficult to see the edges of these areas. The shadowing has been described as 'fluffy' in appearance.
- There is **no loss of volume,** unlike atelectasis, as there is no lung collapse (Fig. 5.11).

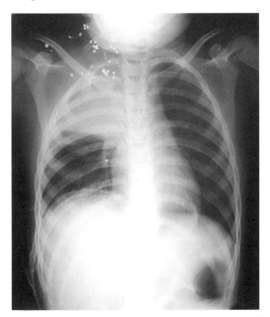

Figure 5.11 Traumatic consolidation of the right upper lobe. There is abnormal whiteness in the right upper lobe. The horizontal fissure is in its normal position, so there is no volume loss. Note the shrapnel in the soft tissues.

- An air **bronchogram** may be seen, particularly when there is extensive consolidation. This is caused by consolidation of lung tissue adjacent to an air-filled bronchus which thus stands out as a black tube amid the consolidative shadowing (Fig. 5.12).

Knowledge of lobar anatomy helps to localize consolidation as it does with atelectasis (Fig. 5.13). It is important in terms of how you treat your patient and may also provide clues as to the cause:

- Aspiration tends to particularly affect the right lower lobe when the patient is erect as the right main and lower lobe bronchi are the most vertical (Fig. 5.14).
- Aspiration is particularly seen in the apical segments of the lower lobes when the patient is supine as these bronchi are directed posteriorly and are thus the most dependent in a patient lying flat.
- Lung contusion tends to occur in the setting of trauma so there may be skin bruising and you may see rib fractures on the CXR (Fig. 5.15).

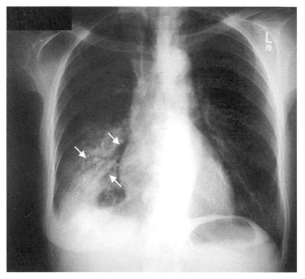

Figure 5.12 Right lower lobe consolidation. The abnormal whiteness in the right lower and mid-zones is poorly defined and 'cloudy'. There is a trident-shaped lucency which is an air bronchogram (arrows). The right heart border remains visible.

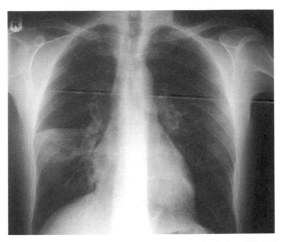

Figure 5.13 Middle lobe consolidation. The poorly defined 'fluffy' increased whiteness abuts the horizontal fissure and there is no volume loss.

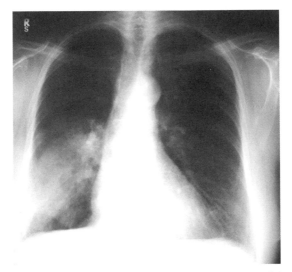

Figure 5.14 Right lower lobe consolidation. The upper limit of this abnormal whiteness shows the location of the apical segment of the right lower lobe, which is in the mid-zone.

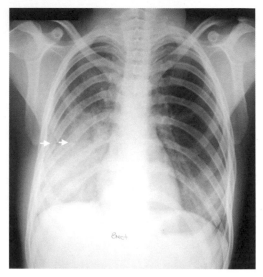

Figure 5.15 Traumatic right lower lobe consolidation. Note the rib fractures (arrows).

- In alveolar pulmonary oedema, the consolidation appearance tends to be situated in the mid-zones around the hila.

In children, infective consolidation is often circular in shape. This is termed a round pneumonia (Fig. 5.16).

> **Remember:**
> In real life, consolidation and atelectasis commonly occur together, but by analysing the abnormal white areas on the CXR you will find that one of these tends to predominate and thus is probably the most important when it comes to treating the patient.

PLEURAL EFFUSION

This refers to fluid in the pleural space. It occupies the dependent part of the pleural space due to gravity so when the patient is erect or semi-erect it occupies the lower zone on CXR initially. However, if the patient is supine, it occupies the posterior surface of the pleural space.

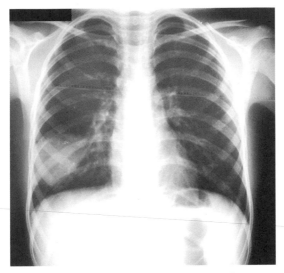

Figure 5.16 Round pneumonia. The rounded patchy white area in the right lower zone represents consolidation.

Radiological Appearance

The characteristic feature of the abnormal whiteness in pleural effusion is that it is **uniform** throughout. It is not patchy.

Most patients that you will see will have their X-rays taken erect or semi-erect:

- A small effusion presents as blunting of the costophrenic angle, the region on the CXR between the hemidiaphragm and the chest wall.
- In a moderate-sized effusion, the top of the fluid is seen as a horizontal line and there is a meniscus at the point where the fluid touches the chest wall. The hemidiaphragm is obscured (Fig. 5.17).
- With a very large effusion there may be shift of the mediastinum away from the side of the effusion. A large effusion is another cause for a 'white-out' appearance but the position of the mediastinum tells you if it is due to atelectasis or effusion (Fig. 5.18).

If the patient is supine the fluid adopts a posterior location. Thus there will be a generalized increased whiteness of the lung field. The lung can still be seen and is effectively being viewed through a thin layer of fluid.

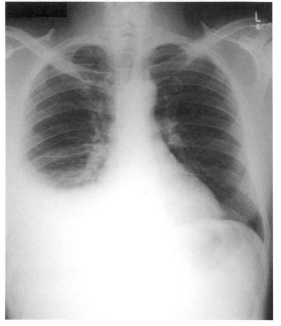

Figure 5.17 Right pleural effusion. There is uniform whiteness at the base of the right hemithorax with a horizontal upper surface and a meniscus seen at the chest wall.

PULMONARY OEDEMA

The majority of cases are due to left ventricular failure. The features are:

- The heart is usually enlarged.
- There may be consolidation around the hila as described above (Fig. 5.19).
- There may be tiny, thin horizontal lines which are seen in the lower zones where the lung touches the chest wall. These are due to oedema in the lung substance or interstitium rather than the alveoli and are known as Kerley B lines (Figs 5.20 and 5.21).
- There are large distended veins seen in the upper zones (Fig. 5.20).
- There may be pleural effusions.

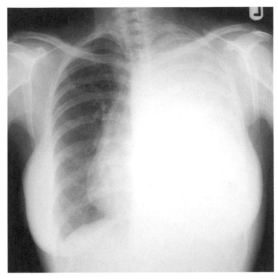

Figure 5.18 Left pleural effusion. There is uniform whiteness over the left hemithorax and the heart and mediastinum are displaced to the right. Thus there is 'too much volume' on the left due to a massive pleural effusion.

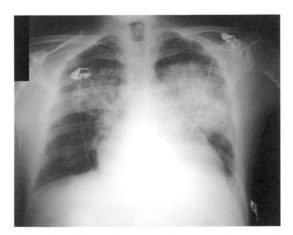

Figure 5.19 Heart failure and alveolar pulmonary oedema. The heart is enlarged and there is bilateral consolidation around the hila, the so-called 'bat's wing' appearance. Note the small left pleural effusion.

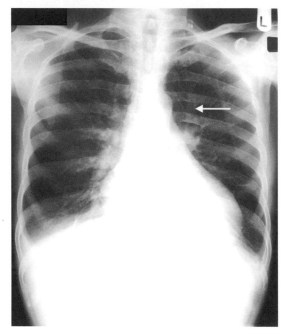

Figure 5.20 Interstitial pulmonary oedema. The heart is enlarged. There is prominence of the upper lobe veins (arrow), representing upper lobe blood diversion. Kerley B lines are seen at the right base and there is a small right-sided pleural effusion.

PNEUMOTHORAX

This is an important cause of a lung field appearing **too black** and refers to air in the pleural space. The features on the CXR are:

- The lung edge is seen as a white line parallel to the chest wall (Fig. 5.22).
- Lung markings do not extend out beyond this white line.
- The area outside this lung edge is blacker than the area inside the line.

A pneumothorax may involve the entire hemithorax and in this case there will be no lung markings visible at all. In a tension pneumothorax the air in the pleural space steadily increases and can build up significant pressure, pushing the mediastinum away towards the

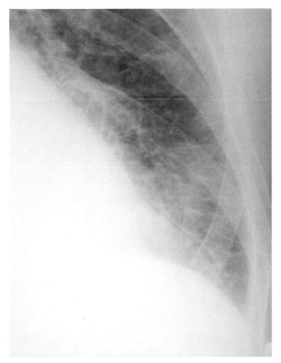

Figure 5.21 Kerley B lines. Thin horizontal white lines are seen reaching the pleural surface at the costophrenic angle.

opposite side (Fig. 5.23). This can cause cardiac arrest and is thus a surgical emergency.

Hazard:
You should not use positive pressure ventilation (e.g. CPAP, IPPB or NIV) in a patient with a pneumothorax as you may turn it into a tension pneumothorax.

Occasionally, the air in the pleural cavity may be located anteriorly, particularly when the patient is supine. This makes it more difficult to see as there may not be a visible lung edge. Be suspicious if the CXR

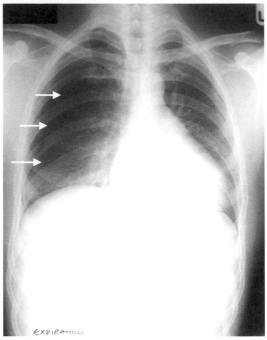

EXPIRATION

Figure 5.22 Right pneumothorax. A black area in the right hemithorax surrounds the right lung, whose edge is clearly seen as a white line (arrows). Lung markings do not extend into this black area.

of a ventilated patient shows one lung to be blacker than the other, particularly in the lower zone, and is associated with otherwise unexplained suboptimal gas exchange.

COPD

The lungs appear hyperinflated and blacker in emphysema due to the destruction of lung tissue. Thin-walled sacs or bullae may develop and appear as particularly black areas, often at the top of the lung. In these cases, unlike pneumothorax, there is no visible lung edge and lung markings are seen reaching the chest wall (Fig. 5.24).

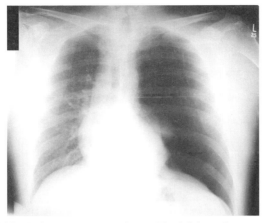

Figure 5.23 Left tension pneumothorax. The left hemithorax contains no lung markings at all. The heart and mediastinum are shifted to the right.

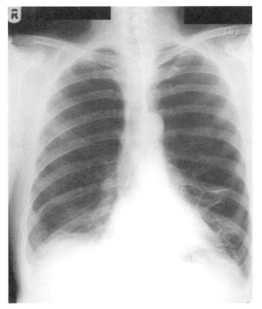

Figure 5.24 COPD. Both lungs are blacker than normal, particularly in the upper zones. No lung edge is visible. Close inspection shows lung markings reaching all the way to the pleural surface and chest wall on each side.

Hazard:
If you use positive pressure ventilation in these patients, be aware that there is a risk of creating a pneumothorax by bursting one of the thin-walled bullae. Usually the benefits to the patient outweigh this small risk but it is important to discuss this with a doctor.

This chapter is a guide to help you interpret abnormal CXRs when on call. However, it is important to develop a systematic approach to reading a CXR so as to obtain all the information available to you.

Acknowledgements

I am grateful to Dr D.J. Delany and Dr I.W. Brown for the use of their extensive film collection and to Dr J.D. Argent for supplying the film of round pneumonia.

Further reading

Corne J, Carroll M, Brown I, Delany D (2002) Chest X-ray made easy, 2nd edn. London: Churchill Livingstone.

POTENTIAL PROBLEMS

The management of sputum retention

Ruth Wakeman

This chapter considers the main causes of sputum retention and offers suggestions for effective and appropriate treatment.

CLINICAL SIGNS OF SPUTUM RETENTION

These are listed in Table 6.1. Note that the patient may present with one or more of these signs.

Table 6.1 Clinical signs of sputum retention[a]

Patient	Clinical signs of sputum retention
Adult	• Increased work of breathing
	• Auscultation: crackles (particularly on inspiration); wheeze; bronchial breath sounds; reduced or absent breath sounds
	• Secretions – audible or palpable
	• Audible secretions or coarse wheeze on cough or huff
	• ↓Oxygen saturations or PaO_2 (hypoxaemia)
	• ↑$PaCO_2$ (hypercapnia)
	• CXR shows patchy shadowing, atelectasis, areas of collapse or air bronchograms
	• Infection: a. ↑Temperature b. ↑HR (tachycardia) c. Elevated inflammatory markers, i.e. white cell count (WCC)
	• Patients may describe difficulty clearing secretions with associated clinical deterioration
	• There may also be associated tachycardia, restlessness, or cyanosis
	Ventilated patients (in addition to those above): • ↑Airway pressures if ventilated in volume cycled modes

table continues

Patient	Clinical signs of sputum retention
	• ↓Tidal volumes if pressure cycled modes (consider alternative reasons for these changes) • Secretions on suction, with an associated clinical deterioration. Alternatively secretions may be difficult to access • Occlusion of the airway lumen may prevent introduction of a suction catheter
Child	• See adult section **Additionally:** • Age-related signs of increased work of breathing (Ch. 7) • CXR – focal collapse may be more common than in adults • Coughing on exercise reported by children or carers **Ventilated children:** • Increased peak inspiratory pressure requirements or a reduction in tidal volumes may be noted
Baby	• See adult section **Additionally:** • ↑Respiratory distress, e.g. common examples: a. Subcostal, intercostal or sternal recession b. Nasal flaring c. Increased respiratory rate d. Stridor e. Cyanosis f. Neck extension g. Expiratory grunting h. Tracheal tug • CXR – areas of collapse are relatively common with sputum retention **Ventilated babies:** • As in children • Diminished chest wall movement or 'wiggle' if high frequency oscillatory ventilation is used

[a] The patient may present with one or more of the signs listed.

POTENTIAL CAUSES OF SPUTUM RETENTION

(See figure on p. 81.)

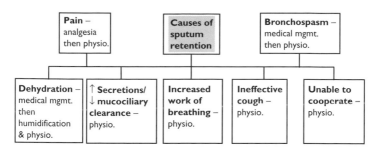

1. EXCESSIVE SECRETIONS ± IMPAIRED MUCOCILIARY CLEARANCE (Table 6.2)

Table 6.2 Treatments and suggested modifications

	Suggested treatment options/modifications
Adult	
Active cycle of breathing technique (ACBT)	• Simple and easily modified. Incorporating thoracic expansion exercises (TEEs), FET and breathing control
Gravity assisted positioning (GAP)	• Modify positioning where poorly tolerated. If mucociliary clearance is impaired (e.g. in primary ciliary dyskinesia) GAP is an important treatment choice
Manual techniques (MT)	• Shaking on expiration may aid sputum clearance. Chest percussion is sometimes used in the clinical setting, the efficacy is unproven
Other treatment modalities	• Patients may already use other techniques, e.g. positive expiratory pressure (PEP), flutter, autogenic drainage or RC Cornet™. It is not appropriate to start a new technique in the on call setting unless you are skilled in its use
Exercise	• Use exercise where tolerated; this complements other airway clearance techniques. Exercise may cause either bronchodilation or bronchoconstriction
Humidification	• Humidify oxygen if at all possible
IPPB	• IPPB is particularly useful where fatigue or work of breathing limit treatment, i.e. the patient cannot take an effective deep breath
Nebulized hypertonic saline (3–7%)	• Hypertonic saline nebulizers can be prescribed for use immediately before airway clearance. It can cause bronchoconstriction;

table continues

	Suggested treatment options/modifications
Inhaled mucolytic drugs, e.g. Pulmozyme	this should be assessed on first use. Hypertonic saline may not be available out of hours • Cystic fibrosis (CF) patients with tenacious secretions may benefit from inhaled mucolytic drugs, e.g. Pulmozyme. The decision to start using this is not generally made in the on call setting. Mucolytic agents such as acetylcysteine may be considered in patient groups other than CF patients
Ventilated adult Gravity assisted positioning (GAP)	• GAP with modifications dependent on cardiovascular or neurological impairment
Manual hyperinflation (MHI)	• MHI can be used to augment lung recruitment and thus mobilize secretions. A fast release on expiration can be employed to mimic a huff or cough; however, the efficacy of this is unproven • An inspiratory hold on the ventilator (if possible) may be useful in those patients unable to tolerate MHI
Suction	• Normal saline is often used clinically to aid clearance of tenacious secretions. Up to 5 ml of 0.9% saline at a time can be instilled via the endotracheal tube or tracheostomy. To date research into the effect of saline instillation remains inconclusive
Humidification	• Humidification is often very useful; consider heated systems • Saline nebulizers can be administered via the ventilator circuit
Manual techniques	• Manual techniques on expiration may assist mobilization of secretions. These can be used in conjunction with MHI or during the expiratory phase of the ventilator cycle
Child ACBT	• As above • From 2–3 years upwards (with blowing games). Progress this to huffing by 3–4 years
Other treatments	• Manual techniques and/or GAP in conjunction with TEEs • Humidification • PEP or flutter may be used at home

	• IPPB (consider pressure settings carefully before use). Generally IPPB is used in children over 6 years
	• Exercise as tolerated
Ventilated child	• As above – GAP, MHI and suction as appropriate
Humidification	• Humidification with or without a heater may prove useful
	• Normal saline is often instilled; the research to date is inconclusive
Bronchoalveolar lavage	• Therapeutic (non-bronchoscopic) lavage could be considered in children, particularly for upper lobe collapse due to sputum plugging. Do not undertake this procedure unless you have been formally trained to use it
Baby	
GAP	• GAP – if children are not yet walking, sitting should be used if the apical segments are affected
Manual techniques	• Clinically, regular position changes and movement appear to be of benefit in mobilizing secretions
	• Infants are unable to participate with TEEs, therefore 30 s percussion with rest periods in between is recommended. This avoids associated desaturation
	• Shaking and vibrations may not be advisable for self-ventilating babies (see ventilated baby, below)
Suction	• Nasopharyngeal suction if ineffectively coughing
Ventilated baby	
GAP	• GAP as above
Humidification	• Humidification with or without a heater is essential
MHI	• MHI (consider the contraindications and precautions discussed in Ch. 18)
Suction	• Suction to clear the secretions
Manual techniques	• Manual techniques can be used. Babies reach functional residual capacity (FRC) at end-expiration. With techniques on expiration it is important to avoid causing collapse – MHI to ↑ tidal volume may be helpful

table continues

	Suggested treatment options/modifications
	• Saline instillation is useful in clearing secretions from tubes <3.0 mm in width
	Modifications for the fatigued patient with increased work of breathing
Adult	
Breathing control	• Incorporate additional breathing control and frequent recovery periods during treatment
Positioning	• Positioning to ↓ the work of breathing and encourage upper chest relaxation, e.g. forward-lean sitting or high side-lying. Aim for a comfortable position where the upper limbs and/or chest are well supported
	• Optimize V/Q match and thus improve oxygenation using positioning (in spontaneously ventilating adults try to position the more affected lung up)
IPPB	• IPPB (high flow rates may be required with very SOB patients)
	• Reassurance is essential
Oxygen	• Appropriate oxygen therapy should be discussed with medical staff
	• Without altering FiO_2 changes in oxygen delivery method can help to relieve SOB. Try using a face mask for mouth breathing patients. Venturi system masks allow delivery of high flow air and oxygen mixtures even for a relatively low FiO_2. The aim is to provide a higher gas flow rate than the patient's inspiratory flow
Positive pressure	• IPPB or NIV can reduce WOB and rest the patient. ACBT with NIV in situ is similar to normal, the inspiratory pressure or time can be increased slightly on the ventilator for TEEs, similar to using IPPB
	• CPAP can reduce WOB. CPAP should be used with care if patients are very fatigued and/or at risk of retaining CO_2 (discuss with the medical team). Secretions can become more tenacious. In clinical practice patients may also find it difficult to regularly remove the mask and expectorate. Regular

	disconnection is detrimental to the benefits gained with CPAP
Other issues	• The importance of rest and sleep should not be underestimated
	• The sensation of breathlessness can be eased with a fan, or open window
Child	• As above
Positioning	• Positioning (V/Q distribution is different in children)
Positive pressure	• NIV incorporating PEEP may be particularly useful as it improves FRC
	• CPAP
	• IPPB for fatigued children over about 6 years
Baby	
Positioning	• Positioning to optimize V/Q and reduce WOB
CPAP	• CPAP is often useful when a baby shows signs of respiratory distress

2. INEFFECTIVE COUGH (Table 6.3)

Patients with a weak cough find airway clearance difficult and tiring, e.g. patients with:

- neuromuscular disorders
- fatigue
- weak respiratory muscles following prolonged ventilation.

Table 6.3 Treatments and suggested modifications

	Suggested treatment options/modifications
Adult	
Increase tidal volume to increase cough effort	• ACBT modified for the individual. Where NIV is used consider a safe increase in inspiratory pressure for TEEs
GAP	• Some patients tolerate head down or flat positions well whereas others cannot; positions may need modifying. IPPB or NIV may allow the patient to tolerate these more comfortably

table continues

	Suggested treatment options/modifications
Manual techniques	• Shaking and vibrations can be helpful. Chest percussion is sometimes used clinically; however, there is little written evidence of efficacy • Fatigued patients may tolerate shaking on alternate breaths more easily
Assisted cough techniques	• Assisted cough techniques can be performed in supine, side-lying or sitting, as indicated. The force is applied on expiration in the direction of chest wall movement • Movement such as rolling or positioning may facilitate clearance of secretions (particularly in high tone patients, e.g. with cerebral palsy) • IPPB or NIV can be used in conjunction with any of the above • Cough assist machine (if available) provides a deep breath, followed by cough assistance using negative pressure. This is most effective if used in conjunction with coughing and assist techniques • Cough stimulation can facilitate a cough if the techniques above are unsuccessful; however, it is unpleasant and not always effective. Consent – as always – should be obtained. Provided the patient has sufficient cough effort a gentle tracheal rub can be applied in the cricoid cartilage area if you are trained
Suction	• Suction if the patient is sufficiently compromised by secretions. Oropharyngeal suction using a Yankauer sucker can be used. Alternatively oropharyngeal or nasopharyngeal suction may be required. Artificial airways (nasal or oral) can be helpful. Without an airway nasopharyngeal suction is made easier and more tolerable by using water-soluble jelly • The risk/benefit of mini tracheotomy insertion may need to be considered; there may be a local hospital policy in place. Mini tracheotomy allows clearance of secretions,

	usually where nasopharyngeal suction has been found to be beneficial, but is unpleasant for the patient. This should be discussed with the medical team
Effective cough	• Paroxysmal coughing can prevent effective clearance of secretions and lead to fatigue or bronchospasm. Advice regarding control of coughing by modification of positioning and breathing control may be helpful. Some patients find swallowing controls paroxysmal coughing; nose breathing may also help
Ventilated adult	• As above • Assisted cough techniques
Child ACBT, GAP, manual techniques Assisted cough techniques	• See above section • ACBT, GAP and manual techniques (see above) • Assisted cough techniques. Where children have a respiratory rate >40 coordination with expiration can be difficult. Closing volumes are high in children and inspiratory assist (NIV or IPPB) could be helpful • IPPB can be considered generally in children aged 6 or above • NIV, particularly machines incorporating PEEP, can improve tidal volumes • Cough assist machine (if available) can be used in children with neuromuscular disease. Consider the associated precautions and contraindications • High tone children may benefit from physiotherapy techniques to reduce tone
Ventilated child	• As Table 6.2
Baby GAP Manual techniques Suction	• GAP • Intermittent chest percussion. It is important to consider closing volume in small children • Cough stimulation is not recommended in children under 6 months • Nasopharyngeal suction may be required; if possible avoid repeated oropharyngeal suction
Ventilated baby	• See Table 6.2

3. UNABLE TO COOPERATE (Table 6.4)

Patients may be unable actively to participate in treatment. Confusion, drowsiness or reduced level of consciousness may affect patients' ability to clear secretions.

Table 6.4 Treatments and suggested modifications

	Suggested treatment options and modifications
Adult Liaise with medical staff to treat the cause of confusion where possible	• A safe level of oxygen therapy to minimize hypoxaemia ($\downarrow$SpO$_2$) • NIV or ventilation to control hypercapnia ($\uparrow$CO$_2$) • Drowsy postoperatively – drugs such as naloxone are sometimes given to reverse the sedative effects of some analgesia. This will also reduce pain control – ensure alternative medication is prescribed • Confused or disoriented patients need clear and concise explanations. Reassurance during treatment may alleviate anxiety. Minimize distractions where possible, and use appropriate visual prompts
IPPB	• IPPB (where voluntary deep breaths are not achievable). Use a face mask with IPPB if an airtight seal cannot be achieved using a mouthpiece
Manual techniques	• Shaking or vibrations with or without IPPB may be beneficial. Some clinicians advocate chest percussion (the evidence for this is inconclusive) • Rib springing or chest compressions can facilitate greater inspiration in unconscious patients • Neurophysiological facilitation of respiration can be useful in drowsy or unconscious patients. These techniques may increase expansion, alter respiratory rate or facilitate an involuntary cough
Cough assist	• Consider cough stimulation where other techniques are unsuccessful (see Table 6.3) • Suction (see Table 6.3)
Ventilated adult	• Clear explanations are required before and during treatment • Sedation may be necessary to treat fully ventilated patients who are agitated or distressed. Liaise with the intensive care team

Child	• See above
	• It is essential to fully explain why and what you are doing to carers, whose input is often extremely useful
	• Some 'unwilling' children can be treated more effectively if distracted or entertained
Ventilated child	• See above
Baby	*Not applicable as babies rarely cooperate!*

4. DEHYDRATION (Table 6.5)

Dehydration can make secretions increasingly thick and difficult to clear.

Table 6.5 Treatments and suggested modifications

Suggested treatment options and modifications	
Adult	
Hydration	• Systemic hydration is the priority. Encourage patients to maintain a sufficient oral intake. If patients are unable to take adequate oral fluids discuss the need for intravenous fluids with medical staff
Humidification	• Humidify supplemental oxygen. Humidification via nasal cannulae is not thought to have any objective effect. It may return dry medical gas to atmospheric humid levels and thus take away the dry feeling of gas
	• Heated water humidification systems can be used with self-ventilating patients or those on CPAP or NIV
	• Nebulized 0.9% or 'normal' saline solution may be helpful. Sterile water can also be considered; however, this may cause bronchoconstriction
	• Ultrasonic nebulizers (with or without heating) can be useful with tenacious secretions (may not be available on call)
Ventilated adult	• Systemic hydration is the main priority. Heated water humidification systems can be incorporated into the ventilator circuit
	• Saline nebulizers can be administered via the ventilator circuit prior to treatment
Child	• See above section

table continues

	Suggested treatment options and modifications
Baby	• Systemic hydration is essential in babies due to their proportionally higher surface area • Head boxes with humidified gas • Saline nebulizers (see above)
Ventilated baby	• See above section

5. PAIN (Table 6.6)

Table 6.6 Treatments and suggested modifications

	Suggested treatment options and modifications

Adult
Pain control
	• Following assessment liaise with medical staff to ensure diagnosis and optimal management of the underlying cause, e.g.:
	  a. wound/trauma pain
	  b. angina management
	  c. management of a pneumothorax
	• Without adequate pain control clearance of secretions becomes very difficult. Liaise with medical staff to ensure optimal analgesia. Consider less common analgesics such as Entonox with rib fractures. This may only be administered by a trained operator
	• Time physiotherapy intervention with the maximal effect of patient's analgesics
	• Positioning may need modification for comfort
	• Teach postoperative patients wound support techniques for coughing and movement
	• Reassurance and clear explanations regarding treatment and pain control are essential
	• Transcutaneous electrical nerve stimulation (TENS)
	• CPAP, e.g. with rib fractures, may help to alleviate pain by splinting the chest wall
	• IPPB appears to be useful when muscular chest wall pain limits TEEs. IPPB may make inspiration a more passive process

Ventilated patient	• Pain may be difficult to assess in sedated patients. Liaise with nursing and medical staff. Again pain control is the priority

Child	• See above • Liaise with nursing and medical staff to ensure optimal assessment and pain control
Ventilated child	• See above
Baby	• See above • The clinical features of pain can be difficult to observe in babies. Appropriate pain scales are available. Liaise with the nursing and medical staff to ensure effective pain relief.
Ventilated baby	• See above

6. BRONCHOSPASM (Table 6.7)

Table 6.7 Treatments and suggested modifications

	Suggested treatment options and modifications
Adult Management of bronchospasm	• Optimal medical management is essential. Well-controlled bronchospasm may allow the patient to clear secretions independently. Medical measures may include inhaled, nebulized or intravenous bronchodilators. Corticosteroids may be required • Assess inhaler technique where appropriate. Patients who are SOB may find a spacer device helpful • Time any physiotherapy treatment required to coincide with the optimal bronchodilator response • Calm, slow treatments in a comfortable position are essential; avoid repeated coughing, huffing as may worsen bronchospasm • IPPB (consider bronchodilators in the nebulizer section) • Manual techniques may increase bronchospasm • Look out for any signs of fatigue, reducing breath sounds and/or increasing CO_2. Alert medical staff immediately. IPPB or NIV can be very effective in offering some rest; however, this must be discussed with the team to ensure that the deterioration is noted and ICU informed

table continues

	Suggested treatment options and modifications
Ventilated adult	• Instillation of saline could aggravate bronchospasm. It is suggested that if required, saline is warmed prior to gentle instillation • Nebulized bronchodilators can be administered before physiotherapy • If MHI is used treatment should stop if wheeze gets worse
Child	• See above section • IPPB is generally an option for children aged 6 or over
Ventilated child	• See above section
Baby	• Liaise with medical staff to ensure optimal control of bronchospasm • Time any physiotherapy to coincide with the best bronchodilator response • The clinical efficacy of beta$_2$ agonists (i.e. salbutamol and terbutaline) is uncertain in children under 18 months
Ventilated baby	• See above section

Key messages

• The key to effective management is thorough assessment. Identify causes of sputum retention not amenable to physiotherapy and liaise with appropriate members of staff. The experienced medical team can be very helpful in guiding good clinical decision making.

• Identify the underlying cause for sputum retention. Treatment options selected depend on the individual. Determine which techniques are most appropriate (and you are most confident with) and which are contraindicated.

• Be flexible in your approach to treatment, adapting techniques for the individual. Careful re-evaluation will identify any modifications required.

• Selection of simple outcome measures is essential in evaluating treatment. Consider SpO$_2$, respiratory rate or volume of secretions.

• Physiotherapy has an important role in the management of sputum retention. Our input in one situation may be advice, in another, intensive treatment.

CHAPTER
7

The management of volume loss

Bernadette Henderson and Nell Clotworthy

There are many diseases and conditions that reduce lung volume.

An accurate assessment will correctly identify which volumes are affected and why (Fig. 7.1). Treatment should be directed at the cause. Remember that not all lung volume loss is amenable to physiotherapy management.

WHAT IS LOSS OF VOLUME?

Consider these questions:

- Which lung volume is affected (static and/or dynamic lung volumes)?
- Is it generalized or localized?

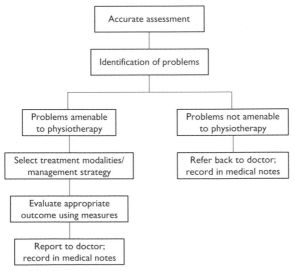

Figure 7.1 Lung volume assessment.

What is Loss of Volume?
- Which lung volume is affected (static or dynamic lung volumes)?
- Is it generalised or localised?
- Is this:
    - a. acute
    - b. chronic
    - c. acute on chronic loss?
- What pathophysiological mechanisms are responsible?

Which Volume is Affected?
In the on call situation the most commonly affected lung volumes are:
- functional residual capacity (FRC)
- tidal volume (TV)
- vital capacity (VC).

Dynamic Lung Volume
Dynamic lung volumes change with respiratory muscle action – i.e. if you want to take a big breath in you can! For example:
- tidal volume (Fig. 7.2)
- vital capacity (Fig. 7.2)

Remember:
Dynamic volume is important for:
- CO_2 clearance
- oxygenation
- the ability to huff or cough effectively.

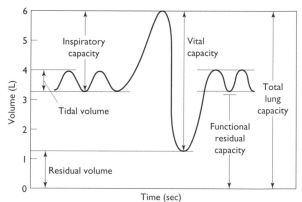

Figure 7.2 Static and dynamic lung volumes. Reproduced with kind permission from Berne and Levy (2000).

Loss of Dynamic Lung Volume

- Loss of dynamic lung volume leads to:
    a. reduction in alveolar ventilation (hypoventilation)

    [Alveolar ventilation = tidal volume (less dead space)
    × respiratory rate]

    b. carbon dioxide retention and respiratory acidosis.
- Hypoxia occurs if alveolar ventilation is reduced and/or metabolic needs of the body are increased.

Static Lung Volume

Static lung volumes do not change with respiratory muscle action – i.e. taking in a big breath cannot increase FRC.

- Functional residual capacity (see Fig. 7.2).

    A loss of FRC may be either generalized or localized:

Generalized Loss of Resting Lung Volume (↓FRC)

There is either:

- increased elastic inward recoil of the lung, e.g. ARDS (the lungs become stiff)
- loss of elastic outward recoil of chest, e.g. kyphoscoliosis

or both.

As FRC decreases towards residual volume a point is reached where dependent airways begin to close (closing volume) (see Fig. 7.3). Gas becomes trapped distal to the closed part of the airway and is rapidly reabsorbed.

Localized Partial or Total Loss of Volume (Collapse or Atelectasis)

There is obstruction of airways at normal lung volume. This results in airway closure and absorption of trapped gases in the lung distal to the obstruction, e.g. sputum retention.

Remember:
Static volume is important to preserve surface area for:
- gas exchange
- V/Q matching
- and therefore oxygenation.

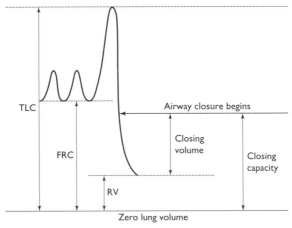

Figure 7.3 Closing volumes. Reproduced with kind permission from Nunn (1999).

Loss of Static Lung Volume

Loss of static lung volume leads to:

- **Reduced lung compliance.**
  a. This increases the work of breathing.
  b. At normal FRC the lungs operate on the steep part of the pressure/volume (compliance) curve – therefore small changes in distending pressure (by the inspiratory muscles) easily produce an increase in volume (see Fig. 7.4a).
  c. At low FRC, lung compliance is reduced (see Fig. 7.4b). Tidal volume is less for the same amount of distending pressure. To produce the same tidal volume at low FRC greater inspiratory muscle effort is required – i.e. breathing is harder work. Collapsed lung needs large distending pressures to reinflate it.

- **Altered length tension in the respiratory muscles.** Muscle has an optimum length for force development. At normal FRC the inspiratory muscles are at their resting length. For a given level of stimulation a muscle produces its maximal force at its resting length. If the muscle length increases or decreases there will be a reduction in the force achieved. With reduced FRC the diaphragm length increases causing a reduction in force generation.

- **Increased airway resistance.** At low lung volumes all air-containing compartments, including the airways, reduce in size. Thus airway resistance increases as lung volume decreases.

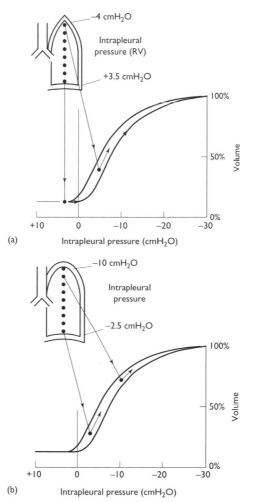

Figure 7.4 Compliance at normal and low lung volume. Reproduced with kind permission from West (1990).

WHY HAS THE PATIENT GOT VOLUME LOSS?

Understanding the underlying pathophysiological mechanisms guarantees appropriate management (Table 7.1).

97

Table 7.1 Underlying pathophysiological mechanisms of volume loss

↓Lung volume due to	Which volume	Cause
Intrusion of abdominal contents into chest	↓FRC	Position, intestinal obstruction, ascites, paralytic ileus, obesity, congenital defect of the diaphragm, diaphragm paralysis
Abnormalities of the pleural space	↓FRC	Pneumothorax, pleural effusion, empyema, haemothorax
Decrease in chest wall compliance	↓TV, FVC, FRC	**Skeletal problems:** a. kyphoscoliosis b. ankylosing spondylitis **Neuromuscular problems:** fatigue due to increased WOB (length-tension inappropriateness); dystrophies; motor neurone disease; myopathies; spinal injuries; cardiovascular accident (stroke)
Airway obstruction	Localized ↓ in volume	Secretions, inflammation, collapse, tumour, oedema, bronchoconstriction, foreign body (**NB paediatrics** – foreign body may cause increase lung volume, i.e. ball valve effect)
Abnormality of lung tissue	Localized ↓ in volume	Pneumonia, consolidation, upper abdominal and cardiothoracic surgery, interstitial lung disease, collapse, ARDS
Loss of respiratory drive	↓TV, FVC	Neurological impairment, excessive narcotic analgesia
Other factors	↓TV, FVC	Pain (incisional/pleuritic, fractures), fear

WORKING OUT THE PROBLEM

The causes of volume loss may mimic one another, making it difficult to identify the real problem.

Table 7.2 lists each of the possible causes together with key assessment 'clues' which should enable the clinician to formulate a working

Table 7.2 Signs and symptoms of volume loss

Condition	History	Chest wall movement	CXR	Arterial blood gases	Auscultation	RR	Lung volume affected	Assessment tool
ARDS/ALI	Many predisposing factors	N/A	Widespread alveolar shadowing	$\downarrow PaO_2$ $\downarrow SpO_2$ $?\uparrow$ $PaCO_2$	Fine inspiratory crackles	$\uparrow$	Static	PaO_2 SpO_2
Consolidation/ pneumonia	Surgery Infection Immobility Aspiration	$?\downarrow$ Over area	$\uparrow$Opacity (whiter) air bronchograms Silhouette sign	$\downarrow PaO_2$ $\downarrow SpO_2$	Bronchial breathing ? Absent BS	$\uparrow$ or N/A	Static	PaO_2 SpO_2 Percussion note
Collapse Generalized dependent atelectasis	Surgery Obesity Prolonged recumbency	$?\downarrow$	Raised hemidiaphragms ? Opacity in the dependent areas	$\downarrow PaO_2$ $\downarrow SpO_2$	$\downarrow$ BS in dependent areas May be bronchial	$\uparrow$ or N/A	Static	Auscultation CXR PaO_2 SpO_2
Collapse Lobar	Surgery Poor cough Pain Incorrect endotracheal tube position	$?\downarrow$ over area	$\uparrow$Opacity Silhouette sign Shift of structures towards opacity	$\downarrow PaO_2$ $\downarrow SpO_2$	Absent BS ? Bronchial breathing if patent airway	$\uparrow$	Static Dynamic	Auscultation CXR PaO_2 SpO_2

table continues

Condition	History	Chest wall movement	CXR	Arterial blood gases	Auscultation	RR	Lung volume affected	Assessment tool
Flail chest	Chest wall trauma/ RTA/fall	Paradoxical	Rib fractures Possible evidence of lung contusion ($\uparrow$opacity)	$\downarrow PaO_2$ $\downarrow SpO_2$	$\downarrow BS$	$\uparrow$	Dynamic Static	PaO_2 SpO_2
Pain	Recent surgery Trauma	$\rightarrow$	Poor inspiratory effort $\downarrow$Lung volumes	$\uparrow PaCO_2$? $\downarrow PaO_2$	$\downarrow BS$	$\uparrow$	Dynamic – leads to static	VAS Observation
Pleural effusion	Recent surgery Malignancy Heart failure Overloaded	Normal May be reduced if large effusion	$\uparrow$Opacity (whiter) Meniscal sign Fluid line if erect film (crisp line if air present)	Normal	$\downarrow BS$	$\uparrow$ if large	Static	CXR Percussion note
Pneumothorax	Trauma Central line insertion Chest drain removed (occasionally caused by drain being	$\rightarrow$ Normal	$\uparrow$Translucency (blacker) May be shift of structures away from translucency Increased definition/	$\downarrow PaO_2$ $\downarrow SaO_2$	$\downarrow BS$ or absent BS Normal (if small)	$\uparrow$	Static	CXR RR PaO_2 SpO_2 Percussion note Subcutaneous emphysema

	put in to drain an effusion) Idiopathic						
Pulmonary oedema	Evidence of heart failure/renal failure/positive fluid balance	N/A	Widespread alveolar shadowing Bilateral hilar flare ? Enlarged heart ? Small effusions seen or fluid in fissures visible	$\downarrow PaO_2$ $\downarrow SpO_2$	Late fine inspiratory crackles +/− wheeze	↑	Static / CXR
Respiratory muscle weakness/fatigue	Medical diagnosis Extensive period of ↑RR Spirometry – FVC↓ Possibly caused by prolonged ventilatory support	↓ ? Paradoxical if phrenic nerve weakness/paralysis	Poor inspiratory effort ↓Lung volumes	$\uparrow PaCO_2$ $?\downarrow PaO_2$ $\downarrow SaO_2$	↓BS	↑ or →	Dynamic Static / $PaCO_2$ FVC

clinical diagnosis. The table also includes a suitable assessment tool for evaluation of treatment success.

Once the clinical diagnosis has been correctly established then the following principles of treatment could apply:

KEY POINTS OF TREATMENT

Table 7.3   Treatment strategies for reduced tidal volume

Aim: To increase tidal volume and decrease respiratory rate
• Breathing exercises: TEE; inspiratory hold; sniff – collateral ventilation (this is not well developed in infants). Infants cannot significantly increase their tidal volumes so will increase their RR to increase their MV • Incentive spirometry. Blowing games: bubbles/windmills, bubble PEP • Neurophysiological facilitation techniques • Mobilization with breathing strategies • IPPB/NIV • Manual hyperinflation where appropriate

Table 7.4   Treatment strategies for reduced FRC

Aim: To increase FRC
• Positioning to optimize FRC, V/Q, diaphragm length tension • CPAP • Increase PEEP • Mobilization with breathing strategies

Table 7.5   Treatment strategies for localized static volume loss, e.g. lobar collapse

Aim: To reverse atelectasis
• Positioning to optimize FRC, V/Q, length tension • Advise regarding optimization of O_2 therapy • Breathing exercises, TEE, inspiratory hold, sniff – collateral ventilation • Incentive spirometry • IPPB • CPAP if good tidal volume • Neurophysiological facilitation techniques • Controlled mobilization • Manual hyperinflation • If secretions present (see Ch. 6)

VOLUME LOSS – MANAGEMENT BY DIAGNOSIS

Table 7.6 Management by diagnosis

Diagnosis	Volume lost	Treatment options	
		Self-ventilating	**Ventilated**
ARDS/acute lung injury	Static Generalized ↓FRC	• Ensure optimization of O_2 therapy • Positioning – erect sitting, side-lying (abdomen free) • CPAP	• Positioning – side-lying (abdomen free), prone • Avoid any manoeuvres which involve disconnecting the patient from the ventilator to preserve PEEP
Consolidation/ pneumonia	Static Localized ↓volume	• Ensure optimization of controlled O_2 therapy. If severe hypoxaemia may require CPAP or NIV • Positioning: Adults – side-lying (abdomen free) with unaffected lung down Paediatrics – side-lying with affected lung down When/if become productive, use airway clearance techniques • Humidification	• Positioning: Adults – side-lying (abdomen free) with unaffected lung down Paediatrics – side-lying with affected lung down • When/if become productive, use sputum clearance techniques • Paediatrics – may tolerate having the affected lung up which would help drain any loose secretions and encourage ventilation to that lung. As in all patients, need to assess individual's tolerance to handling/treatment
Collapse	Static Generalized ↓volume	• Ensure optimization of controlled O_2 therapy. If severe hypoxaemia may require CPAP or NIV • Positioning: Adults – in high sitting (bed or chair), side-lying (abdomen free) Paediatrics – as tolerated and manual techniques/ blowing games in younger patients • Mobilization with breathing strategies	• Recruitment manoeuvres – PEEP, manual hyperinflation ± inspiratory hold • Positioning in high side-lying (abdomen free) • Reverse Trendelenberg (feet down whole bed tilt) • Adults – instillation of 0.9% NaCl Paediatrics – ? selective mini lavage (if trained)

table continues

Diagnosis	Volume lost	Treatment options	
		Self-ventilating	**Ventilated**
Collapse – lobar	Static & dynamic Localized ↓volume	• Ensure optimization of controlled O_2 therapy. If severe hypoxaemia may require CPAP or NIV • Positioning: Adults – side-lying (abdomen free) with unaffected lung down (optimize V/Q & GAP) Paediatrics – side-lying with affected lung down (optimize V/Q) May need to have affected lung up to drain. If poorly tolerated short, frequent treatments. Then when improving may tolerate being left with affected lung up to increase ventilation to that lung • TEEs with inspiratory holds • Neurophysiological facilitation techniques • Incentive spirometry (IS) • IPPB • If in sputum retention use airway clearance techniques	• Positioning: Adults – side-lying (abdomen free) with unaffected lung down (optimize V/Q & GAP) Paediatrics – side-lying with affected lung down (optimize V/Q) • Manual hyperinflation maintaining PEEP • Inspiratory hold • If in sputum retention use airway clearance techniques Paediatrics – selective mini lavage (if trained). If upper lobe problem ? sit up providing ETT well secured
Flail chest	Dynamic Static Localized and/or generalized ↓volume	• Liaise with medical staff to ensure optimal pain control • Ensure optimization of controlled O_2 therapy • Positioning: Adults – side-lying (abdomen free) with unaffected lung down (optimize V/Q) Paediatrics – side-lying with affected lung down (optimize V/Q) • CPAP or NIV to 'splint' the chest wall	• Positioning: Adults – side-lying (abdomen free) with unaffected lung down Paediatrics – side-lying with affected lung down but lying on affected side may be more painful and lead to decreased ventilation (unless patient paralysed and fully ventilated with adequate analgesia) • If in sputum retention use airway clearance techniques

		• TEEs with inspiratory holds • Neurophysiological facilitation techniques • IPPB – avoid use until pneumothorax excluded • If in sputum retention use airway clearance techniques	
Pain	Dynamic Static – generalized ↓volume	• Liaise with medical staff to ensure optimal pain control • Long acting – e.g. PCA Short acting – bolus of opioid, Entonox Regional analgesia • Relaxation techniques • Reassurance	• Lung volumes will not be affected if adequately sedated, analgesed and fully ventilated • If on an assisted mode of ventilation, i.e. pressure support & PEEP then: Liaise with medical staff to ensure optimal pain control Long acting – e.g. PCA if awake Short acting – bolus of opioid • Relaxation techniques • Reassurance
Pleural effusion	Static Dynamic if large	• Positioning: Adults – side-lying (abdomen free) with unaffected lung down (optimize V/Q) Paediatrics – side-lying with affected lung down (optimize V/Q) • NB if pleural effusion very large then the above positioning may cause further volume loss – alter to supported high sitting • Ensure optimization of controlled O_2 therapy • Liaise with medical team ±insertion of inter-costal chest drain (ICD)	• Positioning: Adults – side-lying (abdomen free) with unaffected lung down (optimize V/Q) Paediatrics – side-lying with affected lung down (optimize V/Q) • Liaise with medical team ± insertion of ICD
Pneumothorax	Static – localized	• Liaise with medical team ±insertion of ICD	• Liaise with medical team ± insertion of ICD

table continues

Diagnosis	Volume lost	Treatment options	
		Self-ventilating	**Ventilated**
Pulmonary oedema	Static – generalized	• Ensure optimization of controlled O_2 therapy	• Ensure optimization of controlled O_2 therapy
		• Ensure optimization of controlled O_2 therapy • CPAP • NIV with CPAP facility • Medical treatment • Positioning in high side-lying (abdomen free) Reverse Trendelenberg (feet down whole bed tilt)	• PEEP • Paediatrics – pulmonary oedema may be quite sticky and may potentially cause small airways to block
Respiratory muscle weakness/ fatigue	Dynamic Static – generalized	• Fully supported positioning including shoulder girdle • IPPB • NIV	

Remember:

- Do not apply CPAP if the patient is retaining CO_2 – CPAP does not alter TV and may cause further CO_2 retention and the patient will become $\uparrow$acidotic.
- Consider NIV if patient in type I respiratory failure with a low CO_2 – this may indicate that the patient is working excessively hard, prior to type II respiratory failure.
- Positioning a patient with profound volume loss for treatment may cause desaturation (due to V/Q mismatch) – discuss with the medical team the risk/benefit of increased oxygen while in the position; avoid positions that compromise saturations if supplementary oxygen is not appropriate.

Key messages

- Identify which lung volumes are reduced (see above), and select the strategy which requires the minimum intervention to produce the required outcome.
- Strategies should also include those that can easily be performed by the patient or with the help of the nurse.

Further reading

Berne RM, Levy MN (2000) Principles of physiology, 3rd edn. St Louis: Mosby.

Hough A (2001) Physiotherapy in respiratory care: an evidence-based approach to respiratory and cardiac management, 3rd edn. Cheltenham: Nelson Thornes.

Nunn JF (1999) Nunn's applied respiratory physiology. Oxford: Butterworth–Heinemann.

Pryor JA, Prasad A (2002) Physiotherapy for respiratory and cardiac problems, 3rd edn. London: Churchill Livingstone.

West J (1990) Respiratory physiology. Oxford: Blackwell Publishing.

The management of increased work of breathing

Alison Aldridge

Work of breathing (WOB) = the rate of oxygen consumption of the respiratory muscles.

During quiet respiration:

- The work of breathing is performed entirely by the inspiratory muscles.
- Expiration is passive, powered by the elastic recoil of the tissue.
- As breathing becomes more difficult the muscles work harder and thus the WOB increases.

The efficiency of the respiratory muscles is reduced in patients presenting with:

- respiratory disease
- thoracic deformities
- severe obesity, ascites, pregnancy, etc.
- cardiac disease
- cerebral lesions
- sepsis, etc.

Many patients cope with this reduced respiratory muscle efficiency, until something else happens, e.g. chest infection. This results in a much faster deterioration than normal.

CLINICAL SIGNS (Table 8.1)

Table 8.1 Clinical features of increased work of breathing

	Clinical features of increased work of breathing
Adult (>16 years)	**Respiratory** • ↑RR (dyspnoea) • ↑HR (tachycardia)

	• Mouth breathing
	• Altered depth and pattern of breathing (e.g. deep, shallow, irregular, apnoeas, purse lip breathing)
	• Accessory muscle use
	• Reduced SpO_2
	• Deranged arterial blood gases
	• Carbon dioxide retention (hypercapnia) may cause:
	  a. peripheral vasodilation; warm hands
	  b. bounding pulse
	  c. flapping tremor of hands
	• Secondary signs:
	  a. cerebral – restlessness/irritability/ confusion/seizure/coma
	  b. cardiac – tachycardia/hypertension/ bradycardia/hypotension/cardiac arrest
	  c. fatigue

Child (>2 years)	**Respiratory** The clinical signs are comparable with an adult with the following age-related differences: • ↑RR (tachypnoea) **[2–6 years normal 20–40] [>6 years normal 15–30]** • Intercostal recession • Nasal flaring • Expiratory grunting • Tracheal tug The secondary systemic clinical signs are similar to the adult with the following age-related cardiac differences: • ↑HR (tachycardia) **[Normal 60–140]** • ↑BP (hypertension) **[Normal 95–105/53–66]**
Baby (newborn–2 years)	Respiratory Clinical signs are comparable to a child with the following age-related differences: • ↑RR (tachypnoea) **[newborn normal 30–50 b.p.m.] [<2 years normal 20–40 b.p.m.]** • ↑HR (tachycardia) **[newborn normal 80–200 b.p.m.] [<3 years normal 100–190 b.p.m.]**

table continues

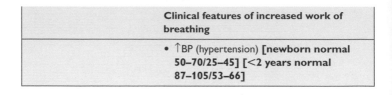

	Clinical features of increased work of breathing
	• ↑BP (hypertension) **[newborn normal 50–70/25–45] [<2 years normal 87–105/53–66]**

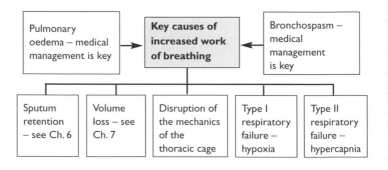

BRONCHOSPASM (Table 8.2)

Bronchospasm is exacerbated by cold, anxiety, dehydration, infection and hypoxia.

Table 8.2 Treatments and suggested modifications

	Suggested treatment options and modifications

Adult	• Check effective bronchodilator therapy, e.g.:
	  a. check technique, regular administration and compliance
	  b. nebulizer therapy requires an adequate tidal volume for effective delivery to the airways – the breathless patient may not receive a therapeutic dose due to small breath size
	  c. intravenous delivery may be more effective (however, potential cardiac side-effects)
	• Use breathlessness positioning to aid relaxation, e.g. forward lean sitting
	• Ensure adequate, controlled oxygen therapy
	• Humidified oxygen therapy
	• Heated humidification if cold system fails to alleviate bronchospasm

- Ensure any retained secretions are cleared effectively (refer to Ch. 6)
- Active cycle of breathing techniques (ACBT). Emphasis upon breathing control, care with FET as the irritability of the airways may lead to spasms of coughing
- Avoid manual techniques, single handed, slow rhythmical percussion can be useful, although evidence is lacking
- Intermittent positive pressure breathing (IPPB):
  a. the system should be set up according to manufacturer's guidelines and local hospital policy and you should only set up and use this equipment if you have been specifically trained and assessed as competent to do so
  b. bronchodilators can be used in the nebulizer
  c. use with high flow rate for patient comfort
  d. try to get patient to rest and let the machine do the work once the breath is triggered

Note: Discontinue immediately if bronchospasm worsens

- Non-invasive ventilation (NIV).
  a. the system should be set up according to manufacturer's guidelines and local hospital policy and you should only set up and use this equipment if you have been specifically trained and assessed as competent to do so
  b. make sure patient comfortable and reassured
  c. let patient hold mask to face before being strapped in so that they feel in control
  d. encourage patient to relax and let the machine help them
  e. you are aiming to rest the respiratory muscles
  f. stay with the patient while they become accustomed to the machine

Note: Discontinue immediately if bronchospasm worsens

- Continuous positive airway pressure (CPAP):
  a. the system should be set up according to manufacturer's guidelines and local hospital policy and you should only set up and use this equipment if you have been specifically trained and assessed as competent to do so
  b. in severe asthma hyperinflation of the lungs is common
  c. in an acute exacerbation, hyperinflation increases as does the WOB
  d. CPAP takes over the effort of maintaining this sustained inspiratory activity and keeps the airways

table continues

Suggested treatment options and modifications	
	open during expiration, thus allowing greater gas emptying
	e. commonly only low pressures are required, 5 cmH$_2$O, and should be prescribed by medical team, as should the required oxygen level
	f. the system should be set up according to manufacturer's guidelines and local hospital policy
	g. a heated humidification system is recommended
Child	• As above
	• Unless using a nebulizer, children between 3 and 5 years are recommended to use an inhaler and spacer, those over 10 years a metered dose inhaler
	• Consider the use of IPPB in the older child (>6 years)
Baby	• As above
	• Bronchodilator therapy. Unless using a nebulizer, children under 2 years are recommended to use an inhaler with spacer and mask
	• Heated humidification is commonly used in the non-intubated baby

DISRUPTION OF THE MECHANICS OF THE THORACIC CAGE (Tables 8.3 and 8.4)

Table 8.3 Disrupted integrity of the thoracic cage

	Suggested treatment options and modifications
Disrupted integrity of the thoracic cage – adult	• Adequate analgesia • Transcutaneous nerve stimulation (TNS) except for cardiac surgery, sternal fractures or patients with pacemakers in situ • Controlled oxygen therapy • Adequate humidification • CPAP to stabilize a flail segment
Disrupted integrity of the thoracic cage – child	• As above, although compliance with CPAP is likely to be poor in younger children • Phrenic nerve damage is a recognized complication post paediatric cardiac surgery resulting in elevation of the diaphragm on the affected side, compression of the lower lobe and persistent collapse

Disrupted integrity of the thoracic cage – baby	• Physiotherapy is directed towards the management of sputum retention (refer to Ch. 6) and postoperative atelectasis (refer to Ch. 12) • As above; however, in infants prolonged ventilation may be necessary and physiotherapy is directed to managing the presenting problems (refer to Ch. 10)

Table 8.4 Respiratory muscle weakness

Respiratory muscle weakness – adult	• Phrenic nerve damage is a recognized complication post cardiac surgery resulting in elevation of the diaphragm on the affected side, compression of the lower lobe and persistent collapse • Neuromuscular weakness affecting the respiratory muscles will gradually present as type II respiratory failure ($\uparrow CO_2$) due to increasing hypoventilation • Inadequate nutrition especially in the presence of a prolonged high metabolic rate (e.g. HIV, cancer) decreases the ability to sustain increased respiratory effort – early ventilatory support is beneficial
Respiratory muscle weakness – child	• As above
Respiratory muscle weakness – baby	• As above

HYPERCAPNIA ($\uparrow PaCO_2$): TYPE II RESPIRATORY FAILURE (Table 8.5)

Refer also to Chapter 11.

Table 8.5 Treatments and suggested modifications

	Suggested treatment options and modifications
Adult	• Hypercapnia $PaCO_2$ >6.0 kPa • Consider treatment options for: a. eliminating the identified cause of the hypoventilation, i.e. sputum retention, bronchospasm, etc. b. managing the cause of the hypoventilation, e.g. thoracic/spinal deformity, muscle weakness, distended abdomen, which leaves the patient unable to compensate for a respiratory problem. Ventilatory support is often needed during the acute illness

table continues

Suggested treatment options and modifications

- Monitor CO_2 and pH regularly. pH below normal levels must be treated – by managing the cause of hypoventilation. Use arterial blood gases or non-invasive transcutaneous CO_2 gas monitoring (if available)
- IPPB. The positive effects of IPPB sessions should be carried over with regular ACBT if possible. You may need to treat the patient little and often. Excellent results are possible with IPPB if NIV is not available to you
- NIV is an effective treatment to increase CO_2 wash out, by increasing tidal volume, if available this must be discussed with the medical team:
  a. the system should be set up according to manufacturer's guidelines and local hospital policy and you should only set up and use this equipment if you have been specifically trained and assessed as competent to do so
  b. check for contraindications
  c. discuss settings with the medical team
  d. correct mask fitting is essential for effective NIV:
     - leave false teeth in situ to maintain normal facial shape and tone
     - watch for leak around NG tubes
     - prevent tissue breakdown on the bridge of the nose, by ensuring good fit
     - avoid air blowing into the eyes
- Set up the machine to the manufacturer's guidelines and local hospital policy
- Consider the need for additional humidification to prevent bronchospasm, secretion retention and further exacerbation of hypercapnia
- Entrain supplemental oxygen through the inspiratory limb of the ventilator in preference to a side port on the mask, and measure with an oxygen analyser
- Set the required minimum respiratory rate in case of complete apnoea due to oxygen therapy
- Monitor regularly for mask leaks, discomfort, claustrophobia, skin damage and gastric distension
- Discuss a management plan with the nursing staff, including how often to come off for drinks, cough, pressure area care, etc.
- Ensure repeat gases are taken 30–45 minutes after setting up to check effect of settings upon the hypercapnia/acidosis. If no effect check with medical team and change settings in line with agreed local policy

	• Gradually reduce time spent on treatment as indicated by the clinical condition and as independent techniques become more effective at maintaining normal gas exchange
Child	• As above, hypercapnia $PaCO_2$ >6.0 kPa
	• Early detection of mild hypercapnia can be managed by either IPPB or NIV
	• The choice of machine and ventilatory setting should be discussed and agreed with the medical team
	• Close monitoring of CO_2 is essential
	• Severe, acute deterioration will require urgent transfer to the paediatric intensive care unit
	• Treatment planning will then be directed at eliminating the identified cause of the hypoventilation, i.e. sputum retention, bronchospasm, etc. (refer to Chs 10, 16)
Baby	• Hypercapnia $PaCO_2$ >5.0 kPa
	• While some NIV machines are suitable for babies, hypercapnia in the very young requires urgent transfer to the paediatric intensive care unit
	• Treatment planning is comparable to a child, as above

HYPOXIA ($\downarrow O_2$): TYPE I RESPIRATORY FAILURE (Table 8.6)

Refer also to Chapter 11.

Table 8.6 Treatments and suggested modifications

	Suggested treatment options and modifications
Adult	• Treat the cause of the $\downarrow O_2$ (hypoxia)
	• Continuous saturation monitoring and arterial blood gases as indicated. Saturation monitoring requires good peripheral circulation. Be aware that accuracy is limited by movement, ambient light, nail varnish, as well as underlying pathologies, e.g. anaemia, jaundice, poor peripheral circulation, etc.
	• Controlled oxygen therapy to maintain SpO_2 >90%
	• Humidification
	• Positioning to maximize V/Q
	• If PaO_2 remains around 8 kPa despite FiO_2 >0.6 (60%) discuss with medical team. Depending upon assessment findings, consider: a. 100% oxygen, rebreathe bag (remember to close valve to fill bag before use)

table continues

Suggested treatment options and modifications	
	b. IPPB to increase tidal volume (Vt), or
	c. CPAP to maximize functional residual capacity (FRC) and oxygenation
	d. these patients may need to be in a high dependency environment
	e. ensure oxygen is available once CPAP/IPPB is removed
Child	• Continuous saturation monitoring and arterial blood gases as indicated. The medical team must be made aware of any change in condition
	• Controlled oxygen therapy to maintain SpO_2 >90%
	• Nasal cannulae are rarely tolerated in young children
	• If PaO_2 remains <8 kPa despite FiO_2 >0.5 consider CPAP; however, careful consideration must be given to mechanical support depending on the underlying cause and tolerance of the child
Baby	• Monitor as above
	• Controlled oxygen therapy. In very young babies it is preferable to maintain the FiO_2 <0.6 to minimize risks of oxygen toxicity and therapy is discontinued as soon as possible
	• Possible methods of delivery are canopy tent, head box, incubator or mask
	• Heated humidification is essential

VOLUME LOSS (STATIC AND DYNAMIC) (Table 8.7)

Table 8.7 Treatments and suggested modifications

	Suggested treatment options and modifications
Adult	• See chapter on volume loss (Ch. 7)
	• Appropriate positioning is essential
	• Treatment should be directed at the primary cause
Child	• As above
Baby	• As above

Postoperative Respiratory Dysfunction (Table 8.8)

The treatment options assume the patient is self-ventilating. Refer to the appropriate chapters for intubated patients.

Table 8.8 Treatments and suggested modifications

	Suggested treatment options and modifications
Adult	• Adequate analgesia • Positioning to improve functional residual capacity and distribution of ventilation • Early ambulation • Thoracic expansion exercises with emphasis on 3 s 'hold' and inspiratory 'sniff' to increase tidal volume and collateral ventilation • Incentive spirometry • IPPB if tidal volume still reduced despite above therapies • CPAP if PaO_2 and FRC still reduced despite above therapies
Child	• As above, although care with IPPB and CPAP as compliance may be extremely poor
Baby	• Adequate analgesia Encourage positioning through play and normal developmental activities, rolling, prone position, etc. • Blowing games in the older baby to facilitate sputum clearance • Severe dysfunction will require prolonged ventilation and physiotherapy is directed to managing the presenting problems. Refer to Chapter 11.

PULMONARY OEDEMA (Table 8.9)

Although the pathophysiological cause is not remediable to physiotherapy the consequent hypoxemia, dyspnoea, tachypnoea and anxiety may respond to intervention while the pharmacological management takes effect.

Table 8.9 Treatments and suggested modifications

	Suggested treatment options and modifications
Adult	• Controlled oxygen therapy • Positioning • CPAP. Discuss with the medical team the level of PEEP and FiO_2 to be prescribed
Child	• Severe sudden onset of pulmonary oedema will require full ventilatory support and is a medical emergency • Management depends on severity of the pulmonary oedema • In older children with mild oedema the adult options may be considered. However, if the intrapulmonary shunt is large the child, whatever age, will require urgent transfer to intensive care for mechanical ventilatory support
Baby	Usually a medical emergency due to the large intrapulmonary shunt generated

SPUTUM RETENTION

Refer to Chapter 6, on the management of sputum retention.

Key messages

- Physiotherapy has a pivotal role in the management of increased work of breathing.
- In order to problem solve and apply clinical reasoning to treatment planning it is easiest to consider that ventilation is the result of a series of interactions between the central control mechanisms, the respiratory muscles, the skeletal structures they influence and the lung tissue itself.
- An increase in the work of breathing may be caused by dysfunction at any one level but it cannot be analysed in isolation, as respiratory mechanics are dynamic in nature.
- Physiotherapy intervention may be directed at more than one point of the system, as dysfunction at one level may disturb, or be compensated for at other levels.
- The skill is to analyse the major cause of the disruption, based on the presenting clinical features and the results of any relevant clinical investigations, and then decide at which level the chosen treatment will be most effective.

Further reading

Hough A (2001) Physiotherapy in respiratory care: a problem solving approach to respiratory and cardiac management, 3rd edn. Cheltenham: Stanley Thornes.

Prasad SA, Hussey J (1995) Paediatric respiratory care: a guide for physiotherapists and health professionals. London: Chapman & Hall.

Pryor JA, Prasad SA (eds) (2002) Physiotherapy for respiratory and cardiac problems, 3rd edn. London: Churchill Livingstone.

SPECIFIC CLIENT GROUPS

Calls to adult intensive care

CHAPTER 9

Rachel Devlin

Calls to an intensive care unit (ICU) are nerve wracking due to the complexity of the environment, the variety of pathologies encountered and the severity of the patient's condition.

However, it is reassuring to remember that all ICU patients are closely monitored and that there is generally one nurse to each patient. Furthermore ICU nursing staff are highly skilled professionals who can offer a wealth of advice and assistance in an on call situation.

This chapter covers the issues surrounding call outs to:

- non-ventilated critically ill patients
- ventilated critically ill patients.

USEFUL TIPS DURING A CALL OUT TO ICU

- Approach your assessment in the same systematic, logical format as that of a ward patient.
- Use your assessment to identify whether the patient's deterioration has been slow over a number of hours or is an acute episode. This will help you identify potential causes for the patient's problem.
- If you are unfamiliar with a piece of equipment or any terminology used (e.g. ventilator settings), do not hesitate to discuss this with the nursing staff who will be able to explain it to you.
- Prior to using positive pressure adjuncts, e.g. IPPB, check all chest X-rays for evidence of a pneumothorax. There is an increased risk of a pneumothorax following insertion of lines, e.g. CVP line, or after removal of an intercostal chest drain.

Hazard:
- There are many alarms in ICU. **DO NOT** switch them off without checking with the nursing staff.

- Explain all interventions to the patient regardless of their sedation levels, in order to minimize anxiety.
- If you do not feel confident to carry out all aspects of your treatment plan, e.g. manual hyperinflation, ask the nurse to assist you.
- Watch the monitors and ventilator closely, to monitor the patient's response to treatment.
- Always check if individual limits to blood pressure, saturations, etc. have been stipulated by the medical team.
- If a patient is cardiovascularly (CVS) unstable, try one treatment technique at a time and then monitor the blood pressure and heart rate response.
- Observe infection control policies closely due to the risk of cross infection.
- Following extubation, physiotherapy treatment aims to prevent reintubation.

THE AIM OF PHYSIOTHERAPY IN THE ICU

The aim of physiotherapy intervention in the intensive care patient is to:

- improve gaseous exchange
- clear secretions
- improve lung volume
- decrease work of breathing
- where appropriate, prevent reintubation of extubated patients.

Common Problems (Table 9.1)

Table 9.1   Common problems and treatment modifications

Common problem	Treatment modification
Sputum retention (see Ch. 6)	**Self-ventilating patient:** • Treat patient as required for the problems identified on assessment • Mobilization, e.g. sitting out of bed, can be appropriate for some patients regardless of the fact that they are in ICU. However, always discuss this with the nursing/medical team first **Intubated patient:** • Treat patient as required for the problems identified on assessment

	• Agree an ongoing management plan with the nursing staff at the end of treatment
Bronchospasm	**Self-ventilating patient:** • Treat patient as required for the problems identified on assessment • Positioning and relaxation may benefit the patient • Ensure nebulizer prior to treatment **Intubated patient:** • Treat patient as required for the problems identified on assessment • Ensure nebulizer prior to treatment • Careful with manual hyperinflation as it may make bronchospasm worse • If required, warm saline prior to use and instil slowly as it may irritate the airways. Discontinue use if symptoms increase • Avoid vigorous manual techniques and protracted use of percussion modes on special beds as these may exacerbate bronchospasm
Pulmonary oedema	**Self-ventilating patient:** • Physiotherapy of no benefit, therefore liaise with medical team regarding diuretics (e.g. furosemide (frusemide)) • If the patient is in type I respiratory failure ($\downarrow$PaO$_2$) CPAP may be indicated • Positioning may be of limited benefit to decrease work of breathing **Intubated patient:** • As above • Positive end expiratory pressure (PEEP), is useful in type I respiratory failure
Pulmonary embolism/ fat embolism (common following long bone fractures)	**Self-ventilating patient:** • Physiotherapy not indicated • Positioning may be of limited benefit to maximize V/Q matching **Intubated patient:** • As above
Pneumothorax	**Self-ventilating patient:** • Physiotherapy not indicated. Patient will require an intercostal chest drain (ICD). Once ICD in situ

table continues

Common problem	Treatment modification
	positioning, exercise, etc. may help reinflation of the lung – not generally an on call emergency
	NB: Do not use IPPB, CPAP, etc. in the presence of an undrained pneumothorax
	Intubated patient: • Physiotherapy not indicated. Liaise with medical team immediately owing to ventilation causing risk of tension pneumothorax. Patient will require an ICD
Non-functioning ICD (e.g. ICD should bubble in the presence of a pneumothorax)	In the case of both self-ventilating and intubated patients, you should liaise with the medical team as the ICD may be blocked or incorrectly positioned NB: ICD may not swing if on suction (see Ch. 14)
Fatigue	**Self-ventilating patient:** • This is a very common cause of failed extubation. Fatigue must be prevented by adequate rest • Reposition the patient to decrease work of breathing, e.g. forward lean sitting over pillows • IPPB may reduce work of breathing or reduce effort of sputum clearance • CPAP will also reduce work of breathing and improve gas exchange • Excessive fatigue may occur requiring non-invasive ventilation or intubation, therefore this should be discussed with the ICU team
	Intubated patient: • This may occur during weaning • Reposition the patient to decrease work of breathing • Discuss with the medical team the potential need to increase ventilatory support, e.g. increased pressure support

Common Issues (Table 9.2)

Table 9.2   Advice on common issues

Common issues	Advice
Ventilator alarming: decreased tidal volume	• Check ventilator circuit for leaks • Consider sputum plug or bronchospasm

	• Patient may be waking up and resisting ventilation/biting on ETT therefore patient may require increased sedation
	• ETT may have moved or there may be a cuff leak that may require anaesthetic review
Ventilator alarming: decreased minute volume (minute volume = tidal volume × respiratory rate)	• See causes of decreased tidal volume
	• If due to hypoventilation because of excess sedation or apnoeas, liaise with the medical team
Ventilator alarming: increased minute volume	• Patient may have developed increased respiratory rate due to pain, anxiety or fatigue therefore may require analgesia, sedation, reassurance or increased ventilatory support
	• Patient may be more awake and making more respiratory effort
Ventilator alarming: increased peak airway pressure (PAP)	• May be due to a sputum plug or bronchospasm
	• Empty excess water from the ventilator circuit
	• Patient may be coughing or resisting ventilation therefore may require increased sedation
	• Present in interstitial lung disease, e.g. fibrosing alveolitis or acute respiratory distress syndrome (ARDS)
Monitors alarming: decreased blood pressure	• Check with nurse that the trace is reliable; if not a blood pressure cuff should be used by the nurse
	• Check that the intravenous lines are patent; if they are kinked drug delivery, e.g. cardiac support drugs, will be affected
	• May occur following turning of the patient; observe if the BP returns to the baseline measurement. If not, return the patient to supine. If low BP persists the patient may require further medical management, e.g. cardiac support drugs
	• May occur due to a bolus or increase of sedation
	• May be due to excess bleeding
	• May occur during manual hyperinflation (MHI) or vigorous manual techniques; if so, stop, allow patient to settle – BP should recover quickly; if not, discuss further intervention with the ICU nurse. One treatment at a time may be possible

table continues

Common issues	Advice
	or there may be a medical solution to support BP during treatment if needed
Monitors alarming: increased blood pressure	• May occur due to pain or anxiety therefore patient may require analgesia or sedation along with reassurance • Always check what limits have been set for the individual patient
Monitors alarming: increased heart rate	• Check heart rhythm – nursing staff can assist • May be due to pain or anxiety, therefore ensure that the patient has adequate analgesia/sedation and reassurance • Also associated with infection or a decrease in circulating blood volume
Monitors alarming: decreased heart rate	• May be due to medication, e.g. sedatives, betablockers, or to vagal stimulation, e.g. following suction or as a result of movement of the ETT • Discuss further intervention with the nurse
Arrhythmias, e.g. atrial fibrillation (AF)	• If you do not understand the ECG trace, ask the nurse to explain it to you • Ensure that the nurse is aware if the ECG trace changes • May compromise BP therefore patient may require further medical management, e.g. cardiac support drugs
Decreased SpO_2	• Check the reliability of the trace (i.e. the heart rate from the pulse oximeter and ECG trace should match). If poor, relocate the probe, e.g. toes, earlobes • Consider sputum retention, decreased lung volume or V/Q mismatch • Patient may require increased FiO_2

Common Conditions (Table 9.3)

Table 9.3 Advice on common conditions

Common conditions	Advice
ARDS (acute respiratory distress syndrome)/ALI (acute lung injury)	• Lung compliance decreases therefore high ventilatory pressures and high PEEP are required. If PEEP >10 cmH$_2$O or the patient

has high PAP ($>30\,cmH_2O$) MHI is strongly advised against ($>15\,cmH_2O$ PEEP – contraindicated)

- Secretions are not always the main problem. Treatment may consist of positioning only, e.g. prone lying to optimize gaseous exchange
- If secretions become a problem ensure adequate humidification along with other techniques to improve sputum clearance (see Ch. 6)
- Nitric oxide (NO – pulmonary capillary vaso-dilator) may be used to improve oxygenation. The patient is generally very unwell – only use MHI if strongly indicated. A special circuit must be used (ask the nurses to help you)

Unfamiliar ventilation equipment, e.g. high frequency oscillatory ventilation	• Ask the nursing staff to explain and to clarify any precautions/contraindications to treatment
Unilateral lung pathology, e.g. pneumonia	**Self-ventilating patient:** • If sputum is the main problem place the affected lung uppermost • If decreased lung volume is the problem, place the affected lung down as there is greater potential to improve ventilation **Intubated patient:** • Due to the rules of ventilation/perfusion (V/Q), the fully ventilated patient should be positioned with the affected lung uppermost to maintain the SpO_2 • If the affected lung is dependent, desaturation is likely to occur
Sepsis – systemic inflammatory response to infection (SIRS) **[Normal WBC = 4–11 × 10^9/L]**	• CVS instability, e.g. decreased BP, will occur and the patient may require cardiac support drugs or fluid management • Positioning in side-lying or MHI may be contra-indicated as these may further compromise BP • Urine output may decrease leading to fluid overload and pulmonary oedema. This will compromise oxygenation and the patient may require increased FiO_2 and increased PEEP • If there are signs of pulmonary infection, try one treatment at a time, e.g. positioning in side-lying and monitor the patient's CVS response

table continues

Common conditions	Advice
Head injuries, neurosurgery and spinal cord injuries	• See Chapter 13 • Make yourself familiar with your unit policies
Spinal fractures	• See Chapter 13 • **Hazard:** Log rolling only until a full set of spinal films has been performed and the spine cleared; medical staff must document if patient can be positioned in any positions other than supine • Note orthopaedic instructions regarding any peripheral fractures
Rib fractures/flail segment/sternal fractures/lung contusion	• Vital to ensure that the patient has effective pain relief in order to comply with treatment • See Chapter 14
Burns	• Ensure that the patient has effective pain relief and adequate humidification, as secretions may be thick and difficult to clear • Early, regular chest clearance is vital to remove soot, etc. particles from lungs. Soot around nose/mouth on admission suggests inhalation injury causing an inflammatory response which results in oedema and sputum • Patients suffering from large-scale burns require rapid fluid replacement therefore are prone to fluid overload • If stridor occurs seek urgent medical advice from ICU due to risk of airway obstruction • Postural drainage is contraindicated in presence of head/neck oedema • Check local policies with regard to movement and manual techniques over skin grafts. Some units allow once the graft is established providing that the graft is healthy and there is thick padding over the affected area. Check with the on call team covering the specialty which undertook the surgery • Escharotomy of the chest wall; effective chest care is essential – however, analgesia is vital • Burns patients are immunosuppressed therefore it is vital to adhere to infection control policies

	• Many units require that passive movements to affected areas are continued for burns patients at weekends – check local policy
Clotting disorders **[Normal INR = 1.0]** **[Normal Hb = 14.0–18.0 g/100 ml (men) 11.5–15.5 g/100 ml (women)]** **[Normal platelets = 150–400 × 10⁹/L]**	• If INR >1.0 (associated with anticoagulants or liver dysfunction) or in the presence of DIC (disseminated intravascular coagulation), bleeding may occur leading to cardiovascular instability • Secretions may be bloodstained and care should be taken if performing suction to minimize trauma. Manual techniques may be contraindicated • If INR <1.0 there will be a predisposition to clotting, e.g. DVT, PE • A falling platelet count may be a sign of sepsis. Low platelets predispose to bleeding and therefore care should be taken during all interventions to minimize trauma to the patient, e.g. when repositioning the patient
Postoperative patients	• See Chapters 12, 13, 14 • Effective pain relief is essential to ensure patient compliance with treatment • Important to observe surgical instructions regarding positive pressure adjuncts, positioning and mobilization
Respiratory medical patients, e.g. COPD	• See Chapter 11 • Aim to prevent patient fatigue by management of increased work of breathing and sputum retention (see Chs 6 and 8) • NIV may be considered. Setting up of NIV may not be the role of the on call physiotherapist therefore important to be aware of individual hospital policy
Renal failure patients	• See Chapter 11 • A patient may present with respiratory problems, e.g. increased RR, however, blood gas analysis shows that it is a compensatory mechanism for a primary metabolic problem, e.g. acute renal failure • Patient may be admitted for haemofiltration (see section on monitors and equipment – Table 9.7)

table continues

Common conditions	Advice
	• Main problem is commonly pulmonary oedema leading to type I respiratory failure. This may respond to diuretics and CPAP • If evidence of secretion retention, use sputum clearance techniques
Complex underlying pathologies with an uncertain medical treatment response (e.g. some cancers, HIV, any rare/unfamiliar medical conditions)	• It is important not to pre-judge the outcome of ICU stay for these patients • Ask what to expect of the underlying pathology if you have not seen it before or if you do not know what influence it might have on your treatment
When there is a high probability of death	• Keep realistic in your expectations of yourself • Balance the probable benefit of your treatment against the discomfort, time and energy that it may require of the patient • Consider competing demands for time, e.g. family, spiritual, religious needs

THE INTENSIVE CARE UNIT CALL OUT

Table 9.4 What do you need to ask?

	What do you need to ask?
Telephone	• Is the patient self-ventilating or ventilated? • Is this a new or existing patient? • Is this an acute or slow deterioration? • What are the patient's observations, e.g. ABGs? • Is the patient CVS stable? • Has the patient had any recent interventions (e.g. insertion of CVP line)? • Has the patient had a recent CXR? If not, could the patient have a CXR prior to your arrival? • Are pain, bronchospasm, etc. all optimally managed?
From the ward staff	• Is the nurse obtaining any secretions via suction or is the patient expectorating independently? If so, how much and what colour are the secretions? • Does the patient cough on suction? • Is the ETT clear? • How does the patient respond to interventions, e.g. turning or suction? • How awake is the patient (if intubated)?

From the charts/monitors	• Is this an acute event or a slow deterioration? • Is this deterioration associated with a particular event, e.g. repositioning or turning sedation off? • Has this occurred previously? • Is the patient CVS stable? • What intravenous drugs is the patient receiving? • What is the patient's overall/daily fluid balance? • Does the patient have a temperature?
Key assessment points	**Self-ventilating patient:** • Is the patient conscious and able to comply with treatment? • Can the patient cough effectively? • Is the patient fatiguing? What is the patient's respiratory pattern/rate? • Does the patient require intubation and ventilation – i.e. are the blood gases deteriorating **Intubated patient:** • How is the patient intubated? • What is the mode of ventilation? • What is the FiO_2 and level of PEEP? • What equipment/lines are attached to the patient (e.g. haemofiltration)?

Table 9.5 Treatment precautions

Treatment precautions	Explanation
Clotting disorders	• Care with suction in order to minimize trauma and prevent unnecessary bleeding • Discuss positive pressure techniques with the medical team (see Ch. 18)
Pre-oxygenation prior to suction	• Suction can cause hypoxia which may lead to arrhythmias therefore increase O_2 before intervention • Important to monitor heart rate during suction as bradycardia may occur
High ICP/spinal cord injuries/neurosurgical conditions	• See Chapter 13
Suction and positive pressure adjuncts following thoracic surgery	• The anastomosis or bronchial stump may be vulnerable to these interventions therefore check with the surgeon • See Chapter 14

table continues

Treatment precautions	Explanation
CVS instability	• Care with manual hyperinflation and vigorous manual techniques as increased positive pressure within the thorax can impede venous return and compromise BP • BP may also be affected by positioning patient in side-lying

Table 9.6 Treatment contraindications

Treatment contraindications	Explanation
Positive pressure adjuncts in the presence of an undrained pneumothorax	• May lead to a tension pneumothorax which may cause the patient to have a cardiorespiratory arrest
Suction/positive pressure in the presence of a base of skull fracture	• Facial fractures, base of skull fracture and ethmoidal approach (i.e. nasal) for neurosurgery contraindicate nasal suction, and facial mask IPPB, CPAP, etc.

Table 9.7 Monitors and equipment

Monitors and equipment	Explanation
Arterial line – blood pressure monitoring	• Inserted via radial, brachial or dorsalis pedis arteries; care with kinking of lines that will make the trace unreliable • Care when moving the patient due to the risk of disconnection • Liaise with the nursing staff regarding reliability of the trace. Blood pressure cuff may be used for more reliable readings
ECG electrodes – heart rate and rhythm monitoring (see Ch. 4)	• Care with techniques that may disrupt the trace and set off the alarms inappropriately, e.g. manual techniques • IABP – the balloon inflates and deflates according to the ECG trace therefore be careful with manual techniques over the pads

CVP (central venous pressure) line – monitors pressure in the right side of the heart	• Commonly inserted in the neck • Drugs may be administered via the CVP line, e.g. cardiac support drugs. Care not to kink the line during turning as drug delivery may be affected, e.g. leading to decreased blood pressure • Risk of pneumothorax during insertion
Swan–Ganz catheter – invasive cardiac monitoring	• Inserted into the neck or groin • Used for accurate measurements in patients who are CVS unstable • Risk of pneumothorax during insertion
Haemofiltration (HF) – renal failure	• Inserted into the neck or groin • Care not to kink HF lines as will affect the working of the machine, e.g. do not flex the hip beyond 45° • Due to rapid changes in fluid status during HF, patient may be CVS unstable and therefore turning may be poorly tolerated
ICP bolt	• See Chapter 13
Ventilators	• Note mode of intubation, e.g. endotracheal tube (ETT), tracheostomy (may indicate long-term ventilation), nasal ETT (may suggest difficult intubation) • Adults have cuffed ETT; if a patient is able to vocalize or there are audible oral noises, inform the nursing staff as there may be a cuff leak that is compromising ventilation • Closed suction systems may be used in ICU; the nursing staff will explain it to you • Many different modes of ventilation are used, therefore ask the nursing staff to explain the settings to you. The aim is to determine whether the patient is fully ventilated, i.e. making no respiratory effort (e.g. continuous mandatory ventilation), or triggering the ventilator independently (e.g. pressure support). Ask the ICU physiotherapist to outline the common modes used during your on call induction

table continues

Monitors and equipment	Explanation
Non-invasive ventilation (NIV)	• See Chapter 18 • Individual hospital policy will dictate whether you are required to set up NIV in an on call situation. However, you may be asked to treat a patient who is receiving NIV. Your treatment will not differ greatly from treating a patient with IPPB. You must not change the settings if you have not been trained in its use and discussed your plans with the medical team
Continuous positive airways pressure (CPAP)	• Improves oxygenation, decreases work of breathing and improves FRC • A good seal of the mask is required to maintain the required level of CPAP • Important to avoid leaks into the eyes and pressure sores on the nose by good mask positioning • Positive pressure follows the path of least resistance therefore preferential ventilation occurs in the non-dependent lung regions • Used in conjunction with positioning
Intermittent positive pressure breathing (IPPB)	• See Chapter 18 • Used to assist sputum clearance and improve tidal volume • Apply rules for positive pressure described previously

Table 9.8 Medication

Medication	Explanation
Sedation	• E.g. propofol (associated with rapid wakening once discontinued), midazolam, thiopental (longer acting sedation – patients slower to wake)
Muscle relaxants	• E.g. atracurium, vecuronium, pancuronium (patients will not cough during suction)
Analgesia	• E.g. morphine (side-effect of respiratory depression), bupivicaine (via epidural), fentanyl (see Ch. 12)
Bronchodilators	• E.g. aminophylline, salbutamol (see Ch. 12)

Diuretics	• E.g. furosemide (frusemide) (non potassium sparing therefore patient may be prone to arrythmias), mannitol
Inotropes	• E.g. noradrenaline (norepinephrine), adrenaline (epinephrine), dopamine, dobutamine (see Ch. 14)
Antiarrhythmics	• E.g. amiodarone, digoxin (see Ch. 14)

Key messages

- Approach assessment of the ICU patient in the same systematic and logical format that you would use to assess a ward patient.
- Work closely with the nursing and medical staff.
- Communicate the outcome of your assessment and treatment succinctly.
- Don't be afraid to ask questions.
- Don't be scared!

Further reading

Hough A (2001) Physiotherapy in respiratory care, 3rd edn. Cheltenham: Stanley Thornes.

Oh TE (ed) (1998) Intensive care manual, 4th edn. Oxford: Butterworth-Heinemann.

Pryor JA, Prasad SA (eds) (2002) Physiotherapy for respiratory and cardiac problems, 3rd edn. London: Churchill Livingstone.

CHAPTER 10

Calls to paediatric intensive care

Elaine Dhouieb

Paediatric intensive care covers a wide range of conditions and ages from premature neonates to 16-year-olds. Physiotherapists should be aware of continuing lung development into teenage years. Chest clearance should only be used where indicated and careful assessment and discussion with medical and nursing staff is needed. Clinical signs may be much more discreet especially in infants.

Take advantage of skilled medical and nursing staff for help and advice available to you in the intensive care unit (ICU). It may be more difficult to gain the cooperation of a small child in treatment, and consent issues must also be considered. Parents will have 24-h access and in most units will not be asked to leave during treatment. Their needs, fears and anxieties must also be considered.

Table 10.1 Aims of treatment

Aims of treatment	
As in adults:	• Remove secretions • Reinflate areas of atelectasis • Reduce airflow obstruction • Improve gas exchange • Decrease work of breathing

Table 10.2 Inappropriate calls

Potentially inappropriate calls	
As adults Inhaled foreign body	• Physiotherapy may move the object further down the bronchial tree. Do not treat until the child has had bronchoscopy to remove. Then treatment may be appropriate

Epiglottitis, croup, stridor	• Unless the child is intubated physiotherapy techniques may increase swelling and compromise respiration • After extubation do not treat for at least 2 hours or if there is significant stridor
Bronchiolitis	• In a self-ventilating infant with no other underlying condition physiotherapy does not add any benefit to good nursing care of positioning, hydration and suction • The ventilated infant should be assessed and treated if indicated
Whooping cough (pertussis)	• In the acute phase of paroxysmal coughing physiotherapy can initiate coughing which may compromise the child • Only treat if retained secretions and the child is paralysed and sedated • May have retained secretions after acute phase
Extreme prematurity or low birthweight	• See Chapter 17

Table 10.3 Advice on common issues

Common issues	Advice
Airways	• Uncuffed nasal ET tubes are usually used to prevent airway damage • These must be securely anchored to prevent accidental extubation or nasal trauma • If the tube is insecure physiotherapy should not take place until it has been retaped
Mechanical ventilation	• Be familiar with the ventilators used in your unit • Pressure limiting ventilation is used to decrease the risk of barotrauma • In pressure ventilation tidal volume will fall with decreased lung compliance, e.g. secretions. This can be used as an outcome measure
PEEP	• PEEP is usually used to prevent airway closure • Must be maintained during manual hyperinflation
Oxygen	• The risk of desaturation with physiotherapy and suction can be avoided if the child is

table continues

Common issues	Advice
	pre-oxygenated by increasing FiO_2 by 10%. Check with nurses that this is appropriate
	• Infants should be hand bagged with an air oxygen mix to prevent retinopathy of prematurity and lung oxygen toxicity
	• Weaning children who are making respiratory effort should be bagged with an air oxygen mix to prevent loss of respiratory drive by blowing off too much CO_2
Inhaled nitric oxide (NO)	• This is used to specifically lower pulmonary arterial pressure (to improve lung compliance) without effect on systemic pressures
	• Patients must be hand bagged with NO and changeover from ventilator to bag should be quick to prevent swings in pulmonary arterial pressure
	• Closed suction or suction through the bagging system port should be used to prevent leak
High frequency oscillatory ventilation (HFO)	• This ventilates by diffusion and is used where limits of conventional ventilation have been reached. It may prevent barotrauma. As physiotherapy techniques, including manual hyperinflation, work by changing pressure they are not indicated unless there are excess secretions and the patient is stable or until the weaning phase
	• Positioning, humidification and suction are vital
	• Closed circuit suction is used to prevent loss of pressure
Extracorporeal membrane oxygenation (ECMO)	• This is used mainly in designated centres and may be useful especially in neonates
	• If the lungs are being inflated it will be at low pressures
	• Anticoagulants make the infant susceptible to bleeds both pulmonary and cerebral. Great care must be taken with lines when positioning
Weaning	• Weaning in infants is more gradual than in adults due to the anatomical and physiological differences (see Ch. 3)
	• Large amounts of dead space, e.g. in ventilator tubing, may increase work of breathing

	• Patient may be weaned onto nasal short tube or mask CPAP
Non-invasive ventilation	• Patients, especially with neuromuscular conditions, may be weaned from ventilation onto this via a mask or tracheostomy • Also useful as an adjunct to chest clearance

Table 10.4 Treatment precautions

Treatment precautions	
Positioning	• Head down position not used. Infants are particularly prone to reflux and as paediatric ET tubes are generally uncuffed there is no airway protection • Prone positioning decreases the work of breathing, improves gas exchange and is often used. Because of the link with sudden infant death syndrome it should not be used in unmonitored infants • Infants and children who are paralysed and sedated are much easier to move but glide sheets, etc. should still be used in the older child both for their comfort and for staff. Great care must be taken not to damage joints and tissues especially in infants • Nesting and containment positioning are important developmentally for ventilated small infants
Percussion, shaking/vibration	• In paralysed and sedated babies the head should be stabilized to prevent shaking injury to the brain
Manual hyperinflation	• As in adults, manual hyperinflation correctly applied can be an efficient adjunct to chest clearance. In children up to 5 years old, open-ended bags are used to prevent over-inflation • As infants are dependent on PEEP it must be maintained. PEEP higher than 7–10 mmHg can be difficult to replicate and hand bagging is not advised • If unsure ask the nurse to bag for you
Bronchioalveolar lavage (BAL)	• Can be diagnostic or adjunct to physiotherapy • Use as taught if unit policy • May cause decreased lung compliance (patient needs increased ventilation), initially • May be effective in acute alveolar collapse or smoke inhalation in stable patient

CONDITIONS

Patients are admitted to PICU with a wide range of conditions. They may have a wide range of congenital or other underlying conditions to be considered. A proportion of children have severe neurological conditions which predispose them to respiratory complications.

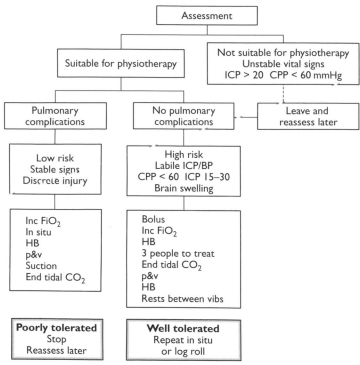

Figure 10.1 To show management of acute paediatric head injury patient. Reproduced with kind permission from Prasad and Tasker (1990).

Table 10.5 Possible conditions

Conditions	
Head injury or cerebral oedema	• See Chapter 13 • See flow chart (Fig. 10.1) • Frequent in children

	• Aim is to prevent secondary injury • May have aspirated at injury • Meticulous assessment – is low cerebral perfusion pressure ($= MAP - ICP$) caused by low BP, neurological (raised ICP) or retained secretions (raised CO_2) • Use three people to treat (bagging, suction and physiotherapy), to prevent swings in CO_2 • Hand bagging may efficiently move secretions with no compromise of CPP • Slow percussion and rests between shaking to prevent stair step (increase with no return to baseline), rise in ICP with increased pressure • Use end tidal CO_2 monitor and manometer in circuit if possible • Assess and treat little but often • When able to turn – log roll to prevent kinking blood vessels and thus reducing cerebral outflow – keep the head in midline • High risk of DVT, use pressure stockings
Cardiac surgery/ cardiology	• Surgery may be palliative (not normal anatomy or blood flow), staging (leading to complete repair) or correcting (normal anatomy and blood flow) • Be aware of change in anatomy and flows (too much or too little blood going to lungs) • If sternum left open, patient is paralysed and at risk of chest problems. Some units treat chest with hand bagging, vibrations and careful positioning
	• Pulmonary hypertensive crisis. Systemic circulation too low to be able to support rise in pulmonary pressure. May be caused by stress or intervention such as physiotherapy, suctioning or retained secretions. Can lead to cardiac arrest. Careful treatment only if retained secretions monitor PA and systemic pressure. Acute treatment MHI with 100% O_2
	• Phrenic nerve damage – raised diaphragm on CXR. Children particularly prone. Loss of lung volume, position head up to reduce work of breathing
Tracheo-oesophageal fistula repair (congenital	• May have a tight repair • No head extension as will stretch the suture line

table continues

hole between trachea and oesophagus)	• No manual hyperinflation unless agreed by team as necessary to clear secretions or inflate atelectasis
	• Careful measured length suction especially when extubated to prevent trauma to repair site
Conditions	
Gastroschisis/ exomphalos (abdominal contents outside wall)	• Distended abdomen • No increase in intrathoracic pressure is allowed, thus care with manual techniques • Manual hyperinflation contraindicated • No manual hyperinflation if lung cysts
Congenital abnormalities of lung	
Diaphragmatic hernia	• Hypoplastic (poorly developed) lung on affected side
	• No manual hyperinflation
Spinal injury (see Ch. 13)	• Surgical repair more rare • Very frightening for young child • Less able to cope with respiratory compromise
Burns	• May use turning bed if artificial skin used (unable to use manual techniques) • Bronchoalveolar lavage (BAL) if smoke inhalation • Care with suction • See Chapter 9
Meningococcal septicaemia	• May be very unstable • May be on haemofiltration • May have pulmonary oedema or cerebral oedema
	• May have low platelet count – care with physio-therapy (see Ch. 15)
Non-accidental injury	• Usually head injury in PICU • May have other injuries

THE CALL OUT

- Information gathered will be similar to that in adult ICU.
- Once you are in the hospital work closely with the nurse and respect the fact that paediatric ICU nurses are exceptionally skilled at handling these children.
- Ask how the child has responded to interventions, e.g. handling, bagging in recent hours to ensure that you are prepared.

- Ask for assistance with aspects of the treatment that you feel least confident in. They will know that you may find the client group tricky and are there to work with you.
- You will be respected more for admitting where you need help. The ultimate aim is to undertake treatment and maintain the stability of all systems.
- It is essential that you spend time working in this environment during your induction.

Key messages

- Look at other appropriate paediatric and ICU chapters.
- Approach assessment and treatment of the paediatric ICU patient in the same systematic and logical format that you would use to assess any patient.
- Work closely with the experienced nursing and medical staff. If in doubt ask. If you feel out your depth seek more senior physiotherapy advice.
- Paediatric patients are more prone to atelectasis/retained secretions. They will fatigue and/or deteriorate quickly – you will need to respond promptly.
- Always support a baby's head when performing manual techniques.
- Reflect on and discuss on call experiences.
- Don't be scared!

References

Prasad SA, Tasker RC (1990) Guidelines for physiotherapy management of critically ill children with acutely raised ICP. Physiotherapy 76(4): 248–250.

Further reading

Prasad SA, Hussey J (1995) Paediatric respiratory care: a guide for physiotherapists and health professionals. London: Chapman & Hall.

Pryor JA, Prasad SA (2002) Physiotherapy for respiratory and cardiac problems, 3rd edn. Edinburgh: Churchill Livingstone.

Calls to the medical unit

Sarah Keilty

This chapter covers:

- Key points to consider when treating medical patients.
- Problem solving respiratory failure to establish the underlying cause, enabling accurate treatment strategies to be put in place.
- Management of patients who are hypoxaemic, hypercapnic and in respiratory distress.

INTRODUCTION

Patients on medical units are often complex. They rarely present with 'single organ failure'. The following may be useful to think about when working through the patient's problems:

- Patients usually exhibit multi pathology.
- As systems are interlinked, if one is compromised another is put under stress.
- The respiratory system is intricately linked to all other major systems, e.g. a primary deficiency in renal or cardiac function will significantly impact on the respiratory system.
- Examine the medical notes with special attention to recent blood, chemistry and laboratory tests as a broader picture of the patient's problems can be gained by assessing renal, liver, and cardiac function.
- Neurological problems are usually related to reduced level of consciousness and ability to protect the airway. Cough depression and risk of aspiration are a serious concern (see Ch. 13).

THE CALL

The primary reasons for calling the physiotherapist urgently to the medical unit are related to respiratory distress, with increased work of breathing and deranged gas exchange. This can be referred to as 'acute respiratory failure'. It may occur with or without the presence of excessive pulmonary secretions and/or sputum retention, and is not necessarily related to a primary respiratory problem. Unrecognized respiratory failure leads to:

- respiratory muscle fatigue
- hypoventilation
- sputum retention
- $\downarrow O_2$ (hypoxaemia).

Accurate assessment to establish the underlying cause is imperative as, if left untreated, it may progress to any or all of the following:

- cardiac arrhythmia
- cerebral hypoxaemia
- respiratory acidosis
- CO_2 narcosis
- coma
- cardiorespiratory arrest.

Thus timely recognition and treatment of acute respiratory failure is of the utmost importance and calling on the physiotherapist for emergency treatment outside usual working hours is an extremely serious part of patient care.

Table 11.1 Types of respiratory failure

Respiratory failure is classified in two categories:
• **Type I respiratory failure:** characterized by the inability to maintain an adequate PaO_2 (hypoxaemia) but the $PaCO_2$ is normal (or slightly reduced)
• **Type II respiratory failure** (ventilatory failure): characterized by a reduced PaO_2 and in addition, the $PaCO_2$ has risen above normal levels (hypercapnia)

HYPOXAEMIA (TYPE I RESPIRATORY FAILURE)

Hypoxaemia = insufficient ability to maintain the PaO_2 above 8 kPa.

Clinical Signs of Hypoxaemia

The clinical signs of a patient with hypoxaemia:

- cyanosis (blue)
- peripherally shut down (cool to touch)

Table 11.2 Classification and causes of hypoxaemia

Classification	Cause
Hypoxic hypoxaemia: • Where blood flows through parts of the lung which are unventilated • Inability to transfer oxygen across the pulmonary membrane (gas diffusion limitation)	• Primary respiratory disease: COPD, pulmonary fibrosis, CF, pneumonia, sputum retention across the thickened (fibrotic/oedematous) respiratory membrane • Primary cardiac disease: heart failure, congestive cardiac failure, pulmonary oedema (causing a diffusion limitation across the respiratory membrane) • Acute bronchoconstriction: asthma (insufficient gas flow in and out of the lung) • Insufficient inspired oxygen therapy (including faulty oxygen delivery equipment)
Ischaemic hypoxaemia: • Usually due to inadequate blood flow through the lung	• Pulmonary embolus • Destruction of the pulmonary vasculature (COPD, pulmonary trauma)
Anaemic hypoxaemia: • Reduction in oxygen carrying capacity of the blood	• Shock (previous significant blood loss with a reduced Hb) • Primary haematological diseases, e.g. sickle cell crisis, anaemia
Toxic hypoxaemia: • Inability for oxygen to be utilized – common in patients admitted with inhalation burns/smoke inhalation injury	• E.g. carbon monoxide poisoning • Cyanide poisoning

• tachypnoea – increased respiratory rate (>20 breaths per minute)
• tachycardia (heart rate >100 b.p.m.)
• low oxygen saturation (<90%)
• confused or agitated if profound hypoxaemia, may not comply with treatment.

Aim of Physiotherapy in Hypoxaemia

- To identify and treat if appropriate the cause of the hypoxaemia, thus aiming to increase the $PaO_2 > 8\,kPa$ while administering appropriate oxygen therapy.

Treatment of Hypoxia

The primary treatment for hypoxia is controlled oxygen therapy, along with identifying and treating the underlying cause.

Table 11.3 Common treatments for hypoxia

Common treatments	Advice
Controlled oxygen therapy	- A drug which should be prescribed as to the required percentage and flow rate - Usually 24–60% can be given by an oxygen mask, humidified or via Venturi system - 24–35% by nasal cannulae; however, a mask is preferable if hypoxaemic and/or mouth breathing - Over 60% oxygen with persistently low sats (<90%) use a non-rebreathe mask to administer constant flow of high concentration oxygen - CPAP is useful with profound hypoxaemia once pneumothorax excluded
Humidification	- Consider cold versus heated humidification - Heated is better for tenacious secretions or severe bronchospasm
Treat the cause, e.g. bronchospasm, sputum retention, volume loss	- If primary respiratory problem treat this - If primary problem is cardiac or renal, discuss your findings with the medical team
Increased work of breathing	- Use airway clearance techniques if needed - Positioning is essential to reduce breathlessness and improve ventilation perfusion matching - IPPB may be useful (with a high flow rate) to rest the muscles and improve efficacy of treatment

Table 11.4 Common issues in hypoxia

Common issues	Advice
Bronchopneumonia	• Ensure medication is optimized (oxygen, analgesia, bronchodilators, antibiotics, etc.) • Positioning to decrease work of breathing • Airway clearance techniques • Humidification
Acute lobar pneumonia	• During the unproductive phase advice on positioning may help reduce WOB • CPAP is useful for hypoxaemia • Sputum clearance is only indicated once the patient becomes productive • *Pneumocystis carinii* pneumonia (PCP – common in immunosuppressed patients, e.g. HIV) presents with profound hypoxia. CPAP is effective; however, pneumothorax is common – CXR is essential
Pulmonary embolus	• Physiotherapy is not indicated. CPAP may help with severe hypoxaemia
Pulmonary fibrosis	• Often present with profound hypoxaemia. Humidified CPAP is effective • Ensure sufficient oxygen is available when CPAP removed
Pulmonary oedema	• CPAP is effective in treatment of pulmonary oedema, left ventricular failure. If very hypotensive, check that BP does not drop with increased intrathoracic pressure – not usually the case
CO_2 retention	• Acute CO_2 retention **is not** a reason to reduce the FiO_2 **unless** patients have evidence of acute-on-chronic CO_2 retention secondary to chronic respiratory disease • This can be diagnosed by correct interpretation of recent blood gas results, assessing pH, in relation to $PaCO_2$, standard bicarbonate and base excess. Only this group of patients require judicious oxygen administration (24–28%), which should be prescribed accordingly

Fatigue	• Hypoxaemic patients may start to fatigue. This is seen by a rising $PaCO_2$ – type II failure. This is an important clinical sign requiring immediate attention. See below
Chronic chest patients	• Patients with longstanding chest disease may have a regular chest clearance routine, e.g. cystic fibrosis, bronchiectatic patients • Discuss this with them and mould your treatment plan to fit their existing regimen and the current physiotherapy problems
Renal failure	• Patients in renal failure may present with ↑WOB • ABGs will show metabolic acidosis, generally with some respiratory compensation – i.e. decreased CO_2 (due to high RR) • Pulmonary oedema and pleural effusion may present
Distended abdomen, e.g. pancreatitis, ascites	• Positioning in alternate side-lying or well supported high side-lying is useful • Standing if possible
Oesophageal varices	• Dilated blood vessels in oesophagus may rupture with increased pressure • Care with coughing, suction contraindicated • Prevent chest infection by positioning, teach huff, mobility if able

HYPERCAPNIA (TYPE II RESPIRATORY FAILURE)

Acute ventilatory failure can be caused by problems in several systems other than the respiratory system. Retention of carbon dioxide reflects hypoventilation. This is caused by a reduction in the extent and efficiency of gas mixing in alveoli and is primarily caused by inadequate alveolar ventilation. Any pathology affecting tidal volume and respiratory rate will affect gas mixing in the alveoli.

A slight rise in CO_2 production will produce a response increasing ventilation by a rise in either respiratory rate, or tidal volume or both. If this response is marked and the respiratory rate is >30/minute the work of breathing is high. The increased muscle work cannot be sustained for long periods and the respiratory muscles begin to

Table 11.5 Causes of acute ventilatory failure

Causes of acute hypoventilation and carbon dioxide retention (acute ventilatory failure)	Explanation
CNS depression	• Opiates used for pain relief, sedation, and drug abuse. Check renal function if on small dose and patient appears drowsy. Tell-tale sign is the presence of small pinprick pupils bilaterally • Alcohol • Head injury
Respiratory disease	• Fatiguing respiratory muscles due to increased work of breathing and a rapid shallow breathing pattern • Poorly functioning respiratory membrane • Oxygen >28% in chronic CO_2 retaining patients
Neuromuscular blockade	• Anaesthesia • Ingestion of poison
Muscle weakness – inability to sustain increased respiratory loads	• Muscle diseases • Fatigue • Long-term steroids • Metabolic abnormalities (renal, liver impairment)
Loss of integrity/restriction of the chest wall – poor pulmonary mechanics	• Pain • Circumferential burns to the thorax • Thoracic trauma • Thoracic cage deformity (kyphoscoliosis) • Previous thoracic surgery
Neurological impairment	• Upper motor neurone lesions (CVA, head injury) may affect respiratory rhythm and pattern • Lower motor neurone lesions (polio, multiple sclerosis, motor neurone disease, etc.) • Neuromuscular junction (myasthenia gravis) • Presenting problems as for muscle weakness (above)

fatigue. If this is the case, patients develop a rapid shallow breathing pattern whereby tidal volume is reduced resulting in an inability to move little more than dead space volume (e.g. 150–200 ml). This means that CO_2 can not be adequately 'washed out' of the lung resulting in CO_2 retention. This causes:

- A surfeit of hydrogen ions producing a respiratory acidosis.
- Agitation and acute confusion.
- These patients may look flushed and peripherally dilated (CO_2 is a potent vasodilator).
- They also may exhibit hand tremor known as CO_2 related 'flap'.
- When CO_2 retention is profound, the patient is drowsy and difficult to rouse and respiratory rate is often reduced (<10 breaths per minute). This is CO_2 narcosis. A likely cause of this is CNS depression.

Treatment of Hypercapnia

Table 11.6 Common treatments for hypercapnia

Common treatments	Advice
Identify and ensure treatment of the *cause* of the hypoventilation	• E.g. if the patient is on an opiate infusion, assessment of the sedation status should be made – especially in elderly patients or patients with reduced renal/liver function as they will not be able to excrete opiates at a normal rate. In discussion with the nursing and medical staff opiate infusions should be reduced or stopped, and reversing agents (e.g. naloxone) administered in severe cases. Alternative pain control should be found • Severe bronchospasm, sputum retention need immediate, careful treatment • If the cause is untreatable, e.g. Guillain–Barré, ventilation must be considered
The primary treatment for acute, severe CO_2 retention is to increase the minute ventilation, without an increase in the total work of breathing	• If respiratory rate is high this can only be achieved by increasing tidal volume. In order to do this assisted ventilation of some form is needed, e.g. IPPB, NIV • IPPB will ↓WOB and ↑TV, thereby ↑O_2 and ↓CO_2, increase efficacy of cough (due

table continues

Common treatments	Advice
	to greater TV) during treatment. NIV will offer the same effect continuously. Do not worry if you do not have access to NIV – IPPB is very effective • If sputum retention is the cause, short regular treatment is invaluable, incorporating IPPB, manual techniques, assisted cough and positioning
Non-invasive ventilation	• Patients who do not respond to the above strategies may retain CO_2 and become acidotic. Non-invasive ventilation (NIV) should be considered in suitable patients, if the resources and training are available in your unit. If not full ventilation will need to be discussed • NIV allows correction of CO_2, acid–base balance by increasing alveolar ventilation. NIV also offloads some of the work of the respiratory muscles, allowing a degree of respiratory muscle rest. NIV is a mode of respiratory support rather than a treatment modality and can be tolerated for protracted periods • Full ventilation has the same effect

Table 11.7 Common issues in hypercapnia

Common issues	Advice
Low pH	• Once pH dips below normal range urgent treatment from the whole team is needed
Call to A&E	• You may be called to resus in A&E as this client group benefit from timely physiotherapy intervention • Do not be scared by this – treat it as a ward, with more help on hand • Start your treatment here
No access to IPPB, CPAP, NIV in ward area	• If a patient requires positive pressure for treatment and no other treatment options

	remain they must be moved to an appropriate area – the medical team should be able to arrange this
• If your hospital does not have access to CPAP, IPPB or NIV treat the patient to the best of your ability using the techniques available to you. Often excellent results are possible. If the patient needs more assistance ICU support will be required – inform the medical staff as to the limitations of your treatment
High probability of death	• If the team establish that death is the most likely outcome the need for treatment must be weighed up against the discomfort felt by the patient and their need to balance the time available against competing demands, e.g. time with family

As suggested, acute ventilatory failure can be caused by problems in several systems other than the respiratory system. However, it is important to stress that it may be caused by an acute deterioration of a chronic condition. It is helpful to read the patient's old notes to establish what the patient's usual status is – see below.

Causes of Chronic CO_2 Retention (Chronic Ventilatory Failure)

Table 11.8 Causes of chronic ventilatory failure

Respiratory disease	• Inadequate alveolar ventilation due to fatiguing respiratory muscles, inadequate surface area for gas exchange
Cardiac disease	• Cardiac failure (LVF/CCF), pulmonary oedema increase respiratory work, with poor oxygenation of the respiratory muscles
Neurological diseases	• Inadequate respiratory muscle strength and endurance
Muscle problems	• As for neurological, above
• Profound malnutrition
• Hyperinflation alongside respiratory disease
Sleep-related breathing disorders	• Severe, longstanding obstructive sleep apnoea, nocturnal hypoventilation/central sleep apnoea

Table 11.9 Common medication effects

Common medication effects	Examples of medication
Bronchodilators	• Nebulized: salbutamol, terbutaline, ipratropium bromide • i.v.: salbutamol, aminophylline
Corticosteroids	• Nebulized: beclometasone • Oral: prednisolone
Diuretics	• Furosemide (frusemide)
Anticoagulants	• Tinzaparin, heparin
Anti-arrhythmics	• Digoxin, amiodarone, adenosine

CALL OUT

Table 11.10 Questions to ask on call out

Specific questions to ask
• What was the patient admitted with, when? • What has led up to the deterioration? • Has the patient had any sedation in the last 12 h? • Has the patient had a recent chest X-ray and arterial blood gas? • Depending upon the presenting problem, can any medication be given prior to your arrival which may help with your treatment, e.g. nebulizers, analgesics, etc.

Arrival

On arrival:

- Look through the medical notes, most recent tests/investigations and recent physiotherapy record.
- Ask what sedation/analgesia the patient has had or whether there are any infusions currently running.
- Try to interpret the CXR – always comparing the most recent film with a previous one if possible. If you are unable to accurately interpret the X-ray, look to see if the most recent CXR appears more abnormal than the previous one. Is the problem bilateral or unilateral? Often, if the shadowing is equal in both lung fields it could be that the problem is systemic, e.g. pulmonary oedema; if it is unilateral or unevenly spread bilaterally it is more likely to be due to a condition affecting the lungs, e.g. consolidation, pleural

disease, fibrosis. There are always exceptions to this rule, so use it as a rough guide! Always check for the presence of a pneumothorax by looking for air in the pleural space.

- Interpret the arterial blood gas – always looking at pH, HCO_3 and base excess in addition to the partial pressures of oxygen and carbon dioxide. By doing this you will be able to decide if the primary problem is respiratory or metabolic. Once you have established this, decide if there is any respiratory or metabolic compensation.

- Examine the patient. If the patient seems very unwell, quickly assess the ABC algorithm (Table 11.11).

Table 11.11 ABC algorithm

A is for airway: Any audible sounds of potential airway obstruction? Can the patient protect the airway? Are there audible secretions, as this means that the secretions are in the upper airway, could potentially obstruct the airway and can be easily obtained with a strong cough or suction
B is for breathing: Respiratory rate, pattern, good tidal volumes? R = L? Accessory muscles? Can the patient talk in complete sentences?
C is for circulation: Colour? Is the patient warm or cold peripherally? Pyrexial? Blood pressure and heart rate and rhythm (regular/irregular, bounding or weak pulse)? Does the patient have a good urine output?
In addition: Is the patient alert? Or does the patient have a reduced conscious level? Or is the patient acutely confused or agitated? Is this new? Has there been a recent neurological event?

Then perform an accurate respiratory assessment, identify the problem(s) and direct treatment accordingly (see tables in above text). Decide on the treatment options you have available to you and then consider the contraindications and precautions. These patients may have multi-pathology, may be cardiovascularly compromised and haemoptysis and pneumothorax are common issues in medical chest patients.

Key messages

- Treatment must be aimed at the cause of the hypoxia and/or hypercapnia so that deranged gas exchange can be corrected and work of breathing reduced.
- Respiratory support in the form of oxygen, positive pressure techniques can support the patient while physiotherapy techniques may expedite recovery.

Further reading

Davidson C, Treacher D (eds) (2002) Respiratory critical care, 1st edn. London: Edward Arnold.

West JB (1995) Respiratory physiology: the essentials, 5th edn. London: Williams & Wilkins.

West JB (1997) Pulmonary pathophysiology: the essentials, 5th edn. London: Williams & Wilkins.

CHAPTER 12 **Calls to the surgical unit**

Valerie Ball

This chapter covers:

- calls to a general surgery patient
- calls to other surgical patients:
  a. vascular surgery
  b. orthopaedic surgery
  c. plastic surgery
  d. ENT and maxillofacial surgery
  e. theatre/recovery
- care of ward-based tracheostomy patient.

CALLS TO A GENERAL SURGICAL PATIENT

This section will concentrate on the problems commonly met by patients having a major abdominal incision (see Appendix 2). The patient may be nursed on a surgical ward or on a high dependency unit, but the principles of management are the same.

Table 12.1 Common problems in patients with abdominal incisions

Common problems	Treatment modifications
Pain	Check drug chart for type/timing of medication: • **All methods** of opiate delivery affect the CNS, cause drowsiness and potentially respiratory depression • **Epidurals** contain less morphine and some include a local anaesthetic; result is less drowsiness and nausea. Nursing staff (within set parameters) can adjust dosage. If not effective needs replacing with an alternative

table continues

Common problems	Treatment modifications
	• **PCA (patient controlled analgesia):** i.v. infusion administered by patient pressing handset. Instruct how to use it – a minute or two before moving/coughing, often misunderstood by patients • **i.m. (intramuscular) morphine** p.r.n.: 4–6 hourly injection, poor pain control from peaks and troughs of delivery – discuss alternatives with medical team if this is contributing to problem • **NSAIDs** and other non-opiates can be requested as an alternative or supplementary if patient is excessively drowsy on morphine; not suitable for all patients • **Alternatives**, e.g. TENS, acupuncture, or Entonox (see below), may be considered but may not be appropriate in call out situation
Unibasal or bibasal atelectasis	• Good positioning • Enlist nurses and family to encourage regular inspiratory breathing techniques, e.g. TEEs with breath hold, end inspiratory sniff
Drowsy patient	• Have analgesia reviewed, e.g. decrease morphine and add NSAIDs to increase alertness (see above)
Weak patient	• Effective positioning • Consider IPPB if poor tidal volume
Pain free, alert patient	• Lean forward sitting on side of bed or in a chair • Stand or mobilize patient (if possible)
Sputum retention	Coughing is required therefore first optimize analgesia, then: • Humidify oxygen immediately (heated is most effective) • Give saline 0.9%, 5–10 ml via a nebulizer if not on humidified oxygen • Position appropriately for drainage but remember it is difficult to cough effectively lying down • ACBT gives the patient control and FET reduces the amount of coughing and its resultant pain • During coughing use wound support with small pillow or folded towel, ideally with the patient sat

up with knees bent up. Some patients find expiratory vibrations on coughing helpful, but avoid manual techniques if they increase pain
- Drips and drains make patients feel very immobile. Teach them how to move comfortably and safely in and out of bed; this is simplest most effective way of mobilizing secretions
- Flutter valves, if used regularly in your unit, empower the patient to continue own treatment
- IPPB with positioning will mobilize secretions well if patient too fatigued to deep breathe
- If secretions are very sticky discuss increasing hydration with medical staff
- Suction (via airway or nasopharygeal)

Criteria for suction:
- All other methods have failed
- Informed consent has been obtained
- Secretions in upper airways
- SpO_2 is dropping

Table 12.2   Common issues in patients with abdominal incisions

Common issues	Advice
Slumped position	• Most common position to find patient with abdominal incision • Use pillows to improve position upright or side-lying as appropriate • Sit patient out of bed as soon as stable
NBM – dry mouth, difficulty expectorating	• Mouth wash positioned where patient can reach it • Use ice cubes/sips of water ONLY if allowed – check with medical staff • Saline nebulizers • Change mask for nasal cannulae if requiring <4 L/min O_2 • Humidify oxygen if requiring mask
Distended abdomen ± paralytic ileus	• Frequently leads to bibasal atelectasis • Position in high side-lying to allow abdomen to fall away from diaphragm • Request medical review to establish cause

CALL OUT

Table 12.3 Questions to ask during the telephone call

What do you need to ask during the telephone call?
• Events leading up to call?
• Type and date of surgery?
• Any limits to mobility, particularly in specialist surgical units?
• Result of any actions already taken?
• Type and effectiveness of pain control?
• Request that analgesia is optimized prior to your arrival

Table 12.4 Questions to ask ward staff

What do you need to ask the ward staff?	Advice
How has patient responded to treatment?	• Any changes while you were en route?
What manual handling implications are there?	• How much assistance will you need if repositioning is required?

Table 12.5 Questions to ask the patient

What do you need to ask the patient?	Advice
Ask patient to move or deep breathe to assess pain control	• If patient can take a deep breath, then most treatment techniques are possible. Ideally patient should be able to move freely in bed and cough
Unable to deep breathe?	• Request an immediate analgesia review. NB: **Intravenous (i.v.) analgesia** will have an almost immediate impact **Intramuscular (i.m.) or oral** will take up to 30 minutes to take effect

Table 12.6 Advice on charts and monitors

Charts/monitor?	Advice
Respiratory rate	• **Low <10** – if due to morphine overdose (patient will often have pinpoint pupils), the patient requires reversal, e.g. Narcan (naloxone hydrochloride). Inform doctor immediately and ensure alternative pain relief prescribed

	• **High >20** – indicating cardiorespiratory compromise (perhaps due to pain, abdominal compromise, volume loss, sputum retention, etc.) or possibly the development of critical illness. A careful assessment is required
Temperature	• **Pyrexia >38.5°C** > 8 hours can be a sign of lower respiratory tract infection. NB: Surgery causes reflex pyrexia when temperature gradually rises and falls within 24 hours of operation – this change in temperature is *not* due to infection
	Raised white blood cell count will confirm infection **[WCC > 11 × 10⁹/L]**
Blood pressure	**High** can be caused by: • Pain/anxiety • Uncontrolled hypertension **Low** can result from: • Dehydration • Postoperative bleeding • Sepsis • Epidural analgesia
Fluid balance: *Normal*	Input: • Is oral intake allowed? • Is i.v. fluid being given? Output: • **[Normal urine output = 1 ml/kg/h]** e.g. a 60 kg woman should pass 60 ml of urine each hour • Include wound drains and insensible loss
Positive balance	Include when calculating: • Blood loss in theatre • A recent history of vomiting and/or diarrhoea • Insensible loss increases by approximately 1 L of fluid for each °C per day above 37°C Look for other signs of fluid retention before assuming a positive balance is fluid overload, i.e.: a. Peripheral pitting oedema b. Frothy sputum c. Dependent fine crackles on auscultation Causes of a positive balance may include: • Left ventricular failure • Cardiac arrhythmia

table continues

Charts/monitor?	Advice
	• Renal failure • Profound malnutrition Remember that pulmonary oedema can coexist with a respiratory tract infection in the severely ill patient
Negative balance	• May be contributing if sputum retention is a problem
O_2 therapy and SpO_2	• O_2 therapy is usually prescribed for 24–48 hours post surgery • Aim to keep **SpO_2 >95%** to reduce the risks of delayed healing, infection and confusion • Patients with pre-existing cardiopulmonary disease may have **nocturnal dips** in SpO_2 for 5 days after surgery
Drug chart	• If **nil by mouth** patient may not have received their usual medication, e.g. a rheumatoid patient, may be more immobile – discuss with team

Table 12.7 Treatment precautions

Treatment precautions	Explanation
Increasing anxiety and pain	• Gaining trust from your patient is vital • Explain the rationale behind your treatment, that **some discomfort is to be expected** when coughing or moving and that you are going to do as much as possible to minimize this • Give patients as much control as possible and **be supportive and careful when moving** or handling them

Table 12.8 Treatment contraindications

Treatment contraindications	Explanation
Postural drainage after gastric surgery	• If cardiac (upper) sphincter of stomach has been removed, anastomosis or oesophagus may be damaged by back flow of gastric contents

Table 12.9 Monitors and equipment

Monitors and equipment	Explanation
PCA via syringe driver	• Handset with wristband which patient ONLY can press to self-administer morphine • Lock out period to prevent overdosing
Epidural via syringe driver	NOT to be disconnected. Careful handling required to avoid dislodging fine bore tube from spinal insertion • Can result in sensory/motor loss in lower limbs limiting mobilization – check limb sensation/movement and use a walking frame for transfers/standing if necessary • Can cause hypotension
Entonox	Can be useful if you are trained in its use (a nurse may be able to administer during treatment) but requires: • Prescribing • Adequate inspiratory effort to activate demand valve • Patient is safe to breathe 50% oxygen/nitrous oxide mix (e.g. no pneumothorax)

CALLS TO OTHER SURGICAL WARD AREAS

Call Out to Vascular Surgery Ward

Table 12.10 Treatment precautions for vascular surgery patients

Treatment precautions	Explanation
Multiple organ involvement associated with peripheral vascular disease	• Often ischaemic heart disease (IHD), cerebral degeneration and/or COPD exist concurrently – adjust treatment to individual needs
Arterial bypass graft viability	Observe when positioning/moving patients for signs of: • Haemorrhage • Thrombosis • Nerve injury causing sensory/motor impairment • Ischaemia below graft site
	Discuss whether mobility is allowed with medical team

Table 12.11 Treatment contraindications for vascular surgery patients

Treatment contraindications	Explanation
Manual techniques over chest wall after axillo-femoral bypass	• Graft passes subcutaneously across chest wall

Call Out to Orthopaedic Surgery Ward

Table 12.12 Treatment precautions for orthopaedic patients

Treatment precautions	Explanation
Osteoporosis	• Particularly common in elderly women. The presence of collapsed thoracic vertebrae restricts chest movement making them highly susceptible to pneumonia after hip fracture • Positioning a patient with a kyphotic chest is challenging, often requiring a compromise between comfort and effectiveness • Manual techniques are contraindicated • Sitting out of bed/mobilizing must be instituted as early as allowed by surgeon
Dislocation of joint replacements	• Discuss with surgeon cost/benefit of positioning for optimal respiratory function
External fixators	• Discuss with surgeon any limits to movement • Positioning a limb with a fixator when requiring side-lying is usually possible by protecting the other limb with pillows • Patients with pelvic fixators may have to remain supine. Physiotherapists have to rely on good instruction in breathing exercises or IPPB to treat effectively
Rib/sternal fractures	See Chapter 14
Spinal injuries	See Chapter 13

Call Out to Plastic Surgery Ward

Table 12.13 Treatment precautions for plastic surgery patients

Treatment precautions	Explanation
Immobilization	• Discuss with surgeon any restrictions in movement

Table 12.14 Treatment contraindications for plastic surgery patients

Treatment contraindications	Explanation
Skin graft viability	• No manual techniques over a graft affecting the chest • Check with nurses the local policy prior to moving patients

Call Out To ENT and Maxillofacial Surgery Ward

Table 12.15 Common problems in ENT and maxillofacial surgery

Common problems	Treatment modifications
Sputum retention following laryngectomy	• Patients have a stoma, a simple hole in the neck • Immediately after surgery blood and exudates may need to be cleared to prevent impairment of respiratory function • Heated humidification is essential • ACBT and FET are possible – wipe secretions away with a suitable sterile swab in the early postoperative stage • Discuss with surgical team before suctioning into the stoma • For tracheostomy tube, see below

Table 12.16 Treatment precautions in ENT and maxillofacial surgery

Treatment precautions	Explanation
Facial reconstruction including flap to mouth	• Discuss with surgeon any protocols which may be specific to the unit (see below for tracheostomy); often the head must be kept in midline

Call Out to Theatre/Recovery

Table 12.17 Common issues in theatre/recovery

Common issues	Advice
Lack of appropriate equipment	• Get patient transferred off trolley onto a bed as soon as possible • Suctioning and oxygen equipment are available but little else – you may need to take humidification equipment with you

Table 12.18 Treatment precautions in theatre/recovery

Treatment precautions	Explanation
Positioning/postural drainage on theatre trolley	• Aspiration at intubation/extubation requires accurate postural drainage aim for best position trolley permits • Drowsy patient, suction immediately

CALL OUT TO WARD-BASED TRACHEOSTOMY PATIENT

Table 12.19 Types of tracheostomy insertion

Surgical tracheostomy	Percutaneous tracheostomy
• Requires theatre conditions • For abnormal anatomy • Tracheal stenosis more common complication	• More rapid procedure • Can be performed in ICU • Stoma heals more quickly on removal of tube

Table 12.20 Types of tracheostomy tube

Type	Usage
Single lumen cuffed tube (see Fig. 12.1)	• Used for invasive ventilation, short-term use <10 days
Double lumen tube cuffed (see Fig. 12.2)	• Used for invasive ventilation, long-term use • Has outer tube fixed with tapes and inner tube which can be removed for cleaning
Double lumen tube uncuffed	• Used when patient's airway is not at risk and not requiring ventilation, for suctioning only
Double lumen tube fenestrated 'FEN' visible on outer flange (cuffed or uncuffed) (see Fig. 12.3)	• A hole in the outer tube which lets air pass over the vocal cords allowing speech when inner cannula is removed/fenestrated inner tube inserted and a cap, speaking valve or finger is placed over the opening
	NB: Take care that unfenestrated tube is in situ before suction
Mini tracheostomy	• Small tracheostomy used for suctioning only; breathing, swallowing and talking are unaffected. Small spigot has to be opened to suction • Is a high risk procedure, therefore the risk/benefit must be considered
Silver tube double lumen	• Permanent tracheostomy

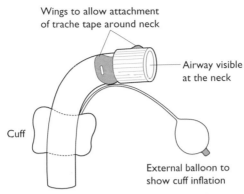

Figure 12.1 Diagram to show single lumen cuffed tracheostomy.

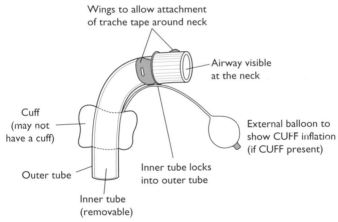

Figure 12.2 Diagram to show double lumen tracheostomy.

The inner cannula in all the double lumen tubes can be removed and should be regularly cleaned/replaced.

Emergency Equipment to be Available at Bedside

A small number of patients with a permanent tracheostomy are admitted for other procedures. Unless they are acutely ill, these patients are generally capable of managing their own tracheostomy. They must, however, have all of the equipment available.

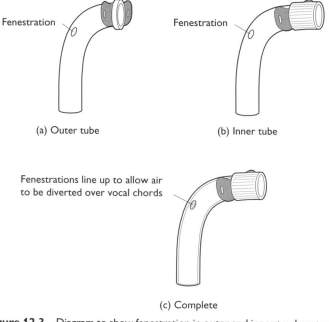

(a) Outer tube   (b) Inner tube

(c) Complete

Figure 12.3 Diagram to show fenestration in outer and inner tracheostomy tubes.

Table 12.21 Emergency equipment

Emergency equipment
• **Tracheal dilator** – to insert into hole and open if tracheostomy tube falls out
• **Spare tracheostomy tubes** (1 same size + 1 size smaller)
• **Spare inner tube** for cleaning purposes (double lumen tubes only) – unfenestrated for suction
• **10 ml syringes**
• **Saline**
• **Humidifier** with O_2 mixing and wide bore tubing or heat and moisture exchanger
• **Tracheostomy mask** (not mini tracheostomy)
• **Suction jar** and tubing
• **Suction catheters** (size to be used = tube size × 2 − 2)
E.g. size 7 tracheostomy tube – 7 × 2 − 2 = size 12 catheter
Mini tracheostomy – size 10 catheter only

- **Gloves and eye protection**
- **Bowl** and access to water for flushing suction tubing
- **Ambu bag** or equivalent with tracheostomy connection

Table 12.22   Common problems in tracheostomy patients

Common problems	Treatment modifications
Sputum plugging in main bronchi	• Ensure humidification equipment is working efficiently. If heated humidifier present, a fan blowing will reduce the temperature and cause condensation in tubing • Obtain sputum specimen if change in sputum indicates a new infection is present • Ensure nursing staff are cleaning/replacing inner cannula (check local protocol for frequency) • If patient is too weak to cough effectively use manual hyperinflation in addition to positioning and manual techniques to mobilize secretions
Excessive secretions	• Assess cause, e.g. a. pulmonary oedema b. new infection, or c. inhalation of saliva (see below) • Ensure patient is not over humidified, after a period of time; the trachea of some patients does not need as much moisture. A heat/moisture exchanger can be used, but the patient needs careful monitoring to prevent sputum thickening and/or plugging
Tube irritation	• Some patients may have a constant cough with minimal secretions, usually due to position of or repeated movement of the tracheostomy tube by humidifier tubing • Discuss best position with patient/carer • Keep suctioning to a minimum • Discuss tube removal if appropriate
Ward staff untrained in tracheostomy care	• You may be looked to for advice. If unsure ask for ICU staff to visit patient

Table 12.23 Common issues in tracheostomy patients

Common issues	Advice
Mini tracheostomy suction difficult/impossible	<ul><li>Secretions too thick to be aspirated by size 10 catheter: a. increase humidification</li><li>Secretions occluding tube: a. insert 2–5 ml 0.9% sodium chloride with syringe b. if all else fails lubricate catheter with sterile jelly</li><li>Wrong catheter being used: a. use size 10 catheters without a beaded end</li></ul>
Saliva/food suctioned from tracheostomy	Uncuffed tube or tube with deflated cuff in patient with impaired swallow reflex can result in saliva or any form of oral intake descending into the trachea:<ul><li>Inflate cuff (use pressure gauge)</li><li>If uncuffed tube issue nil by mouth notice</li><li>Request speech and language assessment as soon as possible</li></ul>
Haemoptysis	<ul><li>Fresh blood will be suctioned from a trachesotomy immediately following insertion and sometimes after a tube change</li></ul>Other causes not related to the above include:<ul><li>High suction pressure. Keep below 20 kPa. If not sure of accuracy of measured pressure in suction tubing, it should just catch a latex glove, not suck it in</li><li>Poor technique of suctioning, not keeping catheter moving or hitting carina</li><li>Not inserting the inner cannula of fenestrated tube can cause trauma to trachea at fenestration point (check inner cannula does not also have a fenestration before suctioning)</li><li>Abnormal clotting – avoid suctioning if possible until stabilized</li></ul>

Hazard:
Totally blocked tracheostomy tube
Thick secretions or blood clot can potentially block the tube.

Signs:
- Rapid deterioration in SpO_2
- Acute respiratory distress
- Cyanosis.

THE PATIENT WILL ASPHYXIATE WITHOUT IMMEDIATE ATTENTION
- Cuffed tube – immediately deflate cuff fully with syringe.
- Double lumen tube – remove inner cannula immediately.
- Single lumen tube – suction immediately to try and clear obstruction.
- Start using ambu bag.
- **If unable to clear call crash team immediately.**

Key messages

- Basal atelectasis is very common after abdominal surgery.
- Dry oxygen exacerbates sputum retention.
- Adequate pain relief is essential before treatment can begin.
- Always check on surgeon's limitations in movement and hydration.

Further reading

Adams et al (1998) The intensive care unit. In: Smith M, Ball V (eds) Cardiovascular/respiratory physiotherapy. London: Mosby.

Hough A (2001) Physiotherapy in respiratory care, 3rd edn. Cheltenham: Stanley Thornes.

Ridey, Heinl-Green (2002) Surgery for adults. In: Pryor JA, Prasad SA (eds) Physiotherapy for respiratory and cardiac problems, 3rd edn. London: Churchill Livingstone.

Singer M, Webb A (1997) Oxford handbook of critical care. Oxford: Oxford University Press.

Calls to the neurology/ neurosurgical unit

Lorraine Clapham

This chapter covers:

- key points to consider in the management of the neurological patient
- the brain injured patient
- the spinal injured patient
- the neuromedical patient.

INTRODUCTION

Disease or injury to the nervous system may affect the rate, pattern and depth of ventilation. Swallow, cough and clearance of secretions may also be affected, which will increase the risk of aspiration pneumonia. On admission to hospital, arterial blood gases may be normal, but respiratory function can deteriorate very quickly, leading to respiratory failure. The physiotherapist needs to be vigilant in the monitoring of these patients. It is important to try to prevent problems and to identify and act upon any deterioration as quickly as possible.

> **Remember:**
> It is usually reduced ventilation and poor airway protection rather than primary lung pathology that causes respiratory failure in these patients.

KEY POINTS TO CONSIDER IN THE MANAGEMENT OF THE NEUROLOGICAL PATIENT

Respiratory management of the neurological patient depends upon:

- airway protection, i.e. maintaining a patent airway
- adequate ventilation.

Features of a Patent Airway
- quiet relaxed breathing
- effective cough capable of clearing secretions
- safe swallow, i.e. no evidence of aspiration (e.g. cough with eat/drink).

If the patient is unable to protect their airway, airway protection techniques will need to be considered.

Airway Protection Techniques
- positioning: on side or recovery position
- manual: chin lift, jaw thrust
- mechanical: oral/nasal airways, cuffed tracheostomy/endotracheal tubes.

Table 13.1 Inadequate ventilation

Features of inadequate ventilation	Result
• Altered respiratory drive • Alveolar hypoventilation • Sputum retention	• $\downarrow O_2$ • $\uparrow CO_2$ • Respiratory failure Type II, i.e. $\uparrow CO_2$ & $\downarrow O_2$
• Aspiration • Respiratory muscle fatigue	• Ventilatory failure

Hazard:
Cerebral oxygenation and oxygenation to other parts of the body is provided by a patent airway. **Occlusion of the airway will result in death.**
WHEN THE LIPS ARE BLUE THE BRAIN IS TOO!

NEUROLOGICAL CONDITIONS

Patients tend to fall into one of three main disease categories:

- brain injury (including surgery)
- spinal cord injury
- peripheral neuropathies and neuromuscular disorders.

Respiratory problems encountered within the same disease category are often similar. However, some groups of patients within a category are considered to be 'high risk' – i.e. clinically less stable – and therefore have more precautions and contraindications associated with their treatment. Common respiratory problems will be considered first followed by an example of the management of a 'high risk' patient from each category.

Brain Injured Patient
- head injury
- cerebral bleed
- cerebral infection
- tumour.

Damage to the brain at the time of injury is irreversible. The aim of treatment is to prevent a secondary cerebral insult leading to further damage, i.e. cerebral ischaemia.

Causes of Secondary Damage
- hypoxaemia – $\downarrow O_2$
- hypercapnea – $\uparrow CO_2$
- hypotension – $\downarrow BP$
- reduced cerebral perfusion pressure (CPP)
- raised intracranial pressure (ICP).

Aim of Treatment
- airway protection
- normal gaseous exchange
- PaO_2 kept above 12 kPa
- $PaCO_2$ normal to low values (4.0–4.5 kPa) if patient is ventilated
- maintenance of CPP above 70 mmHg
- ICP below 20 mmHg.

Aim of Physiotherapy
To maintain or improve gaseous exchange without compromising CPP, which would lead to cerebral ischaemia.

Normal Values
- ICP = intracranial pressure [0–10 mmHg]
- MAP = mean arterial pressure [60–70 mmHg]
- CPP = cerebral perfusion pressure [60–70 mmHg]

E.g. MAP (70) − ICP (10) = CPP (60).

Table 13.2 Common problems in the neurological patient

Common problems	Treatment modification
• Reduced conscious level	• Close 24 h monitoring. Work with nursing colleagues to identify problems and implement treatment plan as appropriate

• Unable to protect airway	• Use airway protection techniques
• Aspiration pneumonia	• Is the patient safe to continue with eating and drinking? Request speech and language therapy referral
• Sputum retention	• Suction • Postural drainage • Chest vibrations/shaking
• Hypoventilation, atelectasis	• Manual hyperinflation • IPPB, NIV **(See precautions for the above)**
• Type II respiratory failure i.e. $\uparrow CO_2 \downarrow O_2$	• Will need anaesthetic opinion, as ventilation may be required

Table 13.3 Common issues in the neurological patient

Common issues	Advice
• High ICP (NB this may be due to respiratory problem, e.g. $\downarrow O_2 \uparrow CO_2$ due to sputum retention and therefore need physiotherapy treatment) • Unstable heamodynamics (may be exacerbated by sedation therefore need to increase cardiovascular support)	• Constantly monitor effects of your intervention • Keep treatment time short • Ensure that respiratory therapy is indicated, e.g. sputum retention. Pulmonary oedema is not an indication for treatment • Nursed head up at 15–35 degrees to reduce ICP (only if they have a protected airway)
• Low CPP. If ICP is raised and blood pressure falls CPP will fall which will cause cerebral ischaemia • Need to modify techniques to minimize effect on ICP, BP and CPP	• Head kept in midline to avoid decreased venous return from the head due to obstruction of neck veins, which will $\uparrow$ICP • When changing patient's position, do so slowly • Tapes securing endotracheal tubes, cervical collars, should not be too tight • Talk to and reassure patient. Explain what you are doing
NB The ventilated patient	• Ensure adequate levels of sedation before start of treatment

table continues

Common issues	Advice
NB Patient with a cerebral bleed, i.e. subarachnoid haemorrhage	• Risk of further bleed, therefore avoid coughing (can be substituted with ACBT and huffing)
	• Caution with activities that affect CVS stability

HEAD INJURED PATIENT: CALL OUT

Common Problems
- Aspiration pneumonia
- Lobar collapse.

Questions To Ask On The Telephone
You need to ask:

- Reason for call out, e.g. aspiration?
- Any other injuries?
- Self-ventilating/ventilated?
- Can they protect their airway?
- Result of ABGs, chest X-ray?
- How stable are they? Cardiovascular, intracranial, i.e. CPP, ICP
- Have parameters been set? – e.g. CPP must be maintained at?
- Precautions/contraindications to treatment, e.g. fracture base of skull (BOS)

Questions to Ask the Ward Staff
You need to ask:

- What is the patient's response to handling/procedures?
- Does **ICP** rise? **CPP** fall? How much? How long does it take to settle? Hopefully almost immediately. If not, risks of treatment will need to be considered.

Information from the Charts and Monitors
- Note observations and any pattern to changes.
- Note if changes relate to changes in patient's position – you may need to avoid these positions.

Your Respiratory Assessment
Establish if treatment is required, e.g.

- sputum retention
- lobar collapse.

Consider risks:
- If ICP is 15 or under with CPP 70 and stable = low risk
- If ICP 15–20 and CPP 70, settles quickly after treatment within 5 minutes = moderate risk
- If ICP 20 + and CPP low = high risk

What Do You Do if the Patient is in the Moderate to High Risk Group but is Severely Hypoxic?

You must be confident that you can improve gaseous exchange by removal of secretions and/or reinflation of collapsed areas. Risk associated with treatment must be minimized. Optimize the situation and proceed with great care. If you are unsure discuss the case with the medical team.

Treatment Precautions

- Manual hyperinflation – low volumes/rate will increase CO_2, and increase ICP. Cardiac output may fall and cause a fall in MAP and CPP – adapt the breath size and speed accordingly.
- Chest vibrations – smooth and gentle – check effect on ICP and CPP.
- Postural drainage – if ICP normal range and stable, patient may tolerate horizontal position; if not, head up position will be required.

Treatment Contraindications

- Head down position – this will increase ICP.
- Nasal airway, nasal suction, NIV, CPAP via a face mask is not permitted for patients with facial or skull base fractures or surgery that involves a transnasal approach, e.g. pituitary tumours.

Monitors and Equipment

- Ventricular drain – permits drainage of cerebrospinal fluid
- Intracranial pressure monitor – records ICP.
- Cerebral function monitoring – CFM.
- Jugular bulb oxygen saturation – indicates cerebral blood flow in relation to cerebral oxygen demand – **[range 50–75%]**.

Surgical Procedures

This may involve drilling, cutting or removing bone, e.g.:

- burr hole
- craniotomy
- craniectomy.

Inserting drains, e.g.:

- wound drains
- CSF drainage, e.g. ventricular drain.

> **Remember:**
> The postoperative management of patients may vary in different neurological units, e.g. to clamp or not clamp ventricular drains when moving a patient. Each procedure will have its own associated precautions and contraindications. You are not expected to know everything. It is essential that you liaise with the staff who are directly involved in the patient's care. They will be able to advise you on what is their unit's current practice. When in doubt discuss with a senior colleague.

SPINAL INJURED PATIENT

Respiratory function in the spinal injured patient is dependent upon the level of the lesion.

Patients with a complete cervical cord injury lose intercostal and abdominal muscle activity and rely on the diaphragm for respiration.

Ascending cord oedema (24–48 h post injury) may result in complete paralysis of the diaphragm.

Table 13.4 Respiratory function is dependent upon the level of the lesion

Level of lesion	Respiratory function
C2	• No respiratory effort
C4	• Partial diaphragm and neck muscles
C6	• Diaphragm and neck muscles
T4	• Diaphragm, some intercostals and neck muscles
T10	• Diaphragm, intercostals, neck and upper abdominal muscles
T12	• Diaphragm, intercostals, neck and abdominal muscles

Table 13.5 Common problems in the spinal injured patient

Common problems	Treatment modifications

• Fear
• Reduced inspiratory/
  expiratory effort
• Atelectasis
• Reduced lung compliance
• Increased work of breathing
	• Reassure patient
	• Positioning – supine may be easier
	  for the tetraplegic patient. IPPB, NIV

• Sputum retention/
  weak cough
	• Change of position will aid drainage of
	  secretions. IPPB, NIV. Assisted cough,
	  suction

• Respiratory muscles fatigue
• Hypoxia, hypercapnia
	• Keep treatment times short. IPPB,
	  NIV may help. Patient may benefit
	  from use of NIV overnight so that
	  they can rest

• Type II respiratory failure	• You will need anaesthetic advice for further management

Table 13.6 Common issues in the spinal injured patient

Common issues	Advice
Injuries above T6 are associated with haemodynamic instability due to loss of sympathetic outflow, resulting in hypotension and bradycardia	• Care with suction procedures – may cause bradycardia and arrest. Availability of i.v. atropine is recommended. Check that the patient has not been fluid overloaded due to over treatment of hypotension
CPAP	• May increase O_2 but will not resolve underventilation and CO_2 retention – use IPPB or NIV

CERVICAL SPINE INJURY: CALL OUT

Questions to Ask on the Telephone

You need to ask about the following:

- The injury – stable or unstable?
- Can the patient be moved?
- Any other injuries?
- Result and time of ABGs?
- Chest X-ray?

- Vital capacity? This is a good indication of respiratory muscle strength. [Normal = 3.5–6 L or 90 ml per kg of body weight]
- Cardiovascular instability? Hypotension, episodes of bradycardia?

Questions to Ask On the Ward

Check again with medical staff:

- level of the injury?
- stability of the injury?
- permission to move the patient?

Information From the Charts

- Note changes in observations, e.g. vital capacity.
- Assess if deterioration was related to change in position.

Your Assessment

- Baseline respiratory assessment.
- Note respiratory effort.
- Breathing pattern.
- Respiratory muscles being used.
- Effectiveness of cough, able to clear secretions.
- Repeat vital capacity measurement.

Treatment Precautions

- Assisted cough, manual techniques – should not be attempted without prior training. Must maintain stability of the spine.
- Suction – may cause cardiac arrhythmia. Need access to i.v. atropine.
- Positive pressure via a facemask may cause abdominal distension.

Treatment Contraindications

- Assisted cough – paralytic ileus, abdominal distension, abdominal injuries.

NEUROMEDICAL PATIENT

Peripheral neuropathies and neuromuscular disorders, e.g.:

- Guillain–Barré syndrome
- Myasthenia gravis.

Early respiratory failure due to neuromuscular paralysis is deceptive. It needs prompt recognition and action. The degree of muscle weakness may not be uniform; there is no correlation between limb power and respiratory muscle power. Patients decompensate rapidly leading to ventilatory failure and respiratory arrest. Anxiety and fear are common.

Table 13.7 Common problems in the neuromedical patient

Common problems	Treatment modifications
• Fear • Breathless, increased respiratory rate	• Reassure patient • Position to reduce the work of breathing • Do not lie patient flat – pressure of abdominal contents against a weak diaphragm can cause respiratory arrest
• Reduced tidal volume • Low vital capacity • Reduced lung compliance • Hypoxia • Respiratory muscle fatigue • CO_2 retention	• NIV, IPPB
• Weak cough • Sputum retention	• Chest vibrations • Increased tidal volume (IPPB, NIV) • Assisted cough • Ensure adequate humidification • Suction
• Autonomic disturbance • Hypotension, tachy/bradycardia, e.g. in Guillain–Barré syndrome	• Care with suction (ensure availability of i.v. atropine)
• Agitation/confusion/unable to cooperate • Respiratory failure • Respiratory arrest	• Seek anaesthetic opinion before this stage is reached • Ventilation will be required

Table 13.8 Common issues in the neuromedical patient

Common issues	Advice
• Patients decompensate rapidly	• Need constant respiratory monitoring O_2, respiratory rate, vital capacity 4-hourly and ABGs if any signs of increasing respiratory distress • Aim to resolve acute episode, and try and prevent recurrence of respiratory problem • Have a **current** treatment and **preventative** action plan

Guillain–Barré Syndrome: Call Out

Common Problems
- hypoxic
  tired!
- retaining secretions.

What do you Need to Ask?
- Did anything precipitate the problem, e.g. lying flat to use bedpan?
- What are the ABGs and vital capacity?
- What position was the patient in when tested?

On the Ward
- Check with staff when deterioration was noted, e.g. after being given a drink? Aspiration?

From the Charts
- Any pattern to deterioration, e.g. reduction in motor power?
- Decline in vital capacity?

Your Assessment
- Baseline respiratory assessment.
- Note position of patient.
- Use of accessory muscles.
- Paradoxical chest movement – chest wall moves out abdominal wall moves in = **weak diaphragm**.
- Quality of voice – nasal, wet, gurgle = pharyngeal weakness and risk of aspiration.
- Quality of cough – is it effective?
- Vital capacity – 1000 ml or below, patient will need to be considered for ventilatory support.

Contraindications
- Do not lie patient flat.

Precautions
- Suction – cardiovascular disturbance, e.g. bradycardia.
- Positive pressure via face mask may cause gastric distension.

Remember:
If respiratory function continues to deteriorate due to the progressive nature of the neuropathy, ventilation may be unavoidable.

Further reading

Harrison P (2000) Systemic effects of spinal cord injury: respiratory system. In: HDU/ICU. Managing spinal injury: critical care. London: Spinal Injuries Association, ch. 12.

Hough A (2001) Disorders in intensive care. In: Hough A (ed.) Physiotherapy in respiratory care: an evidence-based approach to respiratory and cardiac management, 3rd edn. Cheltenham: Stanley Thornes, ch. 15.

Lindsay KW, Bone I, Callander R (1997) Neurology and neurosurgery illustrated, 3rd edn. New York: Churchill Livingstone.

CHAPTER 14 Calls to the cardiothoracic unit

Sarah Boyce

This chapter covers:

- cardiac surgery
- thoracic surgery
- chest trauma.

CARDIAC SURGERY

Types of Cardiac Surgery
- Coronary artery bypass graft (CABG). Taking the grafts from long saphenous vein, internal mammary artery and/or radial artery.
- Mitral valve replacement (MVR).
- Atrial valve replacement (AVR).
- Decoarctation of aorta (resect narrowed area).
- Repair of atrial or ventricular septal defect (ASD, VSD).
- Heart transplant ± heart lung transplant.

These are usually performed through a median sternotomy incision (Appendix 2) while the patient is on cardiac bypass.
Other surgery:

- Transmyocardial revascularization (TMR). Laser channels are formed in the myocardium to increase blood flow to an ischaemic area, access is via a left thoracotomy incision.

Aims of Physiotherapy Treatment
- Prevent sputum retention.
- Optimize lung volume – there will be significant volume loss.
- Early mobilization (usually able to sit out day 1, and sometimes mobilize – check local policy).
- Prevention of shoulder, thoracic stiffness (check your local policy).

Table 14.1 Common problems in cardiac surgery patients

Common problems	Treatment modifications
Pain	• Ensure good analgesia • Reassure patient • Teach wound support • Encourage effective cough • Patients often experience feeling of restricted expansion – reassure and encourage TEEs • Chest drains can increase pain. Reassure that this is temporary and inform nurses to ensure drains come out as soon as appropriate
Lower lobe collapse	• Very common, especially LL lobe due to anaesthetic, deflation and handling of lungs, length of procedure, need for supine lying in theatre, etc. • Usually will recover with very regular, effective positioning, TEEs, using hold/sniff techniques, mobilization, etc. Empower the patient to continue • CPAP can be effective with significant or persistent collapse • Check notes to see if phrenic nerve (stimulates diaphragm) damaged during surgery. This may explain persistent collapse or respiratory failure
Impaired renal function	Usually caused by hypotension May cause: • Pulmonary oedema • Pleural effusion Initially treated with furosemide (frusemide), if not successful a renal dose of dopamine. Severe failure is treated with haemofiltration/dialysis on the ICU
Pulmonary oedema	• Requires medical treatment of the cause • CPAP can be useful to improve SpO_2, reduce work of breathing
Pleural effusion	• Usually requires chest drain insertion • Ensure continued mobility and chest care
Chest infection	• Check if patient has been prescribed antibiotics • Ensure effective, humidified oxygen therapy • Ensure effective sputum clearance
Hypotension	• Possible causes: a. ↓blood volume (hypovolaemia) (secondary to fluid restriction or bleeding)

table continues

Common problems	Treatment modifications
	b. cardiac failure
	c. arrhythmias
	• Discuss with nursing staff; medical therapy may be available to support BP
	• Be aware that positive pressure, e.g. CPAP/MHI, may further reduce BP
	NB: Make sure you know what medical BP therapy is in reserve. This may be needed if treatment compromises BP, if no further BP support possible – proceed with care
	• Patient should not be mobilized if on noradrenaline (norepinephrine) or adrenaline (epinephrine). Always discuss with nurse if considering getting a patient out of bed
Hypertension	• Can cause grafts to rupture
	• Avoid agitating the patient, optimize analgesia, discuss mobility with nursing staff if high systolic (>140 mmHg) or diastolic BP (>90 mmHg)

Table 14.2   Common issues in cardiac surgery patients

Common issues	Advice
Perioperative myocardial infarction	• Check op notes or anaesthetic records • Discuss mobility with surgeons
Arrhythmias	• Ask nurse to help interpret any ECG changes (see Ch. 4) • Most common is atrial fibrillation (see Chapter 4). Always check with nursing staff before mobilizing a patient • If the patient is in AF and HR is very fast this can cause ↓BP – the patient may be clammy and sweaty. Mobility is inappropriate if ↓BP • Usually treated with digoxin • If very severe patient may need to be cardioverted (shocked with a defibrillator to restore sinus rhythm)
Cardiac tamponade	• Increased pressure on heart due to bleeding inside pericardium • Patient needs immediate surgical intervention to prevent cardiac arrest • Signs are ↑HR, ↑CVP with ↓BP

Pneumothorax	• Check CXR; usually requires chest drain
CVA	• Look for signs of neurological deficit; check that the patient has had anticoagulation therapy if appropriate. Advise nursing staff on positioning
Sternal wound complications	• Failure to unite and/or infection • May reduce expansion and cough due to pain and altered mechanics • If possible use mobility to prevent other complications
Patient very agitated postoperatively (known as post-pump delirium)	• May be caused by reduced cerebral perfusion during cardiac bypass • Ensure other reasons for confusion have been ruled out, e.g. hypoxia, renal problems
Heart transplantation	• Treat like all other cardiac surgery • Rejection will require medical management

CARDIAC SURGERY CALL OUT

Table 14.3 What do you need to ask?

Information source	What do you need to ask?
Telephone	• When and what operation? • Has the postoperative recovery been routine? • What signs of chest infection? • Is the patient's CVS stable and if not, how unstable? • Recent CXR? • Is pain control optimized? • What O_2 is the patient receiving, is it sufficient, humidified, has the patient had a nebulizer (if appropriate)? • Can they reposition the patient? Suggest position
From ward staff	• How has patient responded to reposition, etc.? • What is the patient's fluid balance? CVS status? Temperature? • Speed of deterioration?
From charts/ monitors	• Check BP, HR and temperature. Is this supported by medication, is the trend stable? • Saturations (SpO_2)
Key assessment points	• Determine if the problem is cardiac, renal or respiratory in origin

Table 14.4   Treatment precautions

Treatment precautions	Explanation
Positive pressure techniques, e.g. IPPB, CPAP, NIV, MHI	• If BP is low this could further compromise cardiac output • Discuss with nursing staff if anything can be done to support BP, e.g. medication, or if blood volume is low extra fluid may help • Treat slowly changing one thing, e.g. position, MHI, etc., at a time to minimize effect on BP • MHI – intersperse single big breaths with periods of tidal volume breathing
Manual techniques	• If patient has an intra-aortic balloon pump in situ (see p. 189) do not disturb the ECG leads as the machine cycles with the ECG trace • Care with an unstable or infected sternal wound

Table 14.5   Treatment contraindications

Treatment contraindications	Explanation
Positive pressure techniques Sitting patient up with IABP Mobilization/sitting patient out of bed	• If undrained pneumothorax present • Will kink IABP line in femoral artery • If on inotropes (unit policy will differ – check this on induction) • Low BP • IABP/haemofiltration in situ • Medical staff/nurses advise against – check with senior staff if unsure

Table 14.6   Monitoring

Monitoring	Explanation
Mean arterial pressure (MAP) **[65–100 mmHg]**	• Mean perfusion pressure over the complete cardiac cycle
Central venous pressure (CVP) **[3–15 cmH$_2$O]**	• Reflects the functioning of the right side of the heart and the pressure in the venous system • ↑Heart failure, positive fluid balance, increased pressure in thorax (e.g. pneumothorax) • ↓Negative fluid balance

Fluid balance	• Measures fluid in and out • Fluid loss e.g. bleeding, NG drainage, urine output (retention of fluid is common due to poor renal function/↓urine output) • Fluid replacement blood/products and fluids
Left ventricular function	• Usually preoperative studies • Described as poor, moderate or good • If poor postoperatively exercise tolerance will be reduced
Swan–Ganz catheter or transoesophageal Doppler	• Measure complex cardiac functioning – all you need to know is how unstable the patient is to enable you to weigh up the risks of treatment • If Swan–Ganz recently inserted check CXR for apical pneumothorax

Table 14.7 Equipment

Equipment	Explanation
Cough lock (tight band of material fastened around thorax)	• Used if patient has 'clicky'/unstable sternum • Pulled tight when patient coughs • Not to be left tight continuously as limits thoracic expansion
Intra-aortic balloon pump (IABP)	• Used to treat patients who require an immediate reduction in cardiac workload • Access through femoral artery to the ascending aorta. Controlled via the ECG leads (be very cautious with any manual techniques), helium filled balloon inflates during diastole and deflates during systole • Patient not allowed more than 30 degrees hip flexion, to avoid kinking. Can be ¼ turned (hip supported with pillows) if BP tolerates • Care with effect of treatment on BP
Pacing wires	• Temporary pacing wires inserted into myocardium. NB: patient has to lie flat for approximately 1 h post removal of wires, as there is potential for tamponade • Patient can mobilize with pacing box. Note what the underlying rhythm is, e.g. asystole, sinus bradycardia

table continues

Equipment	Explanation
	• If pacing wires come out seek help immediately • If wires become detached from box reconnect straight away and inform nurse
Chest drains	• Usually 2–3 inserted for drainage • Look for any sudden or large amounts of drainage – could indicate bleeding • Prevent shoulder stiffness by regular full range exercises

Table 14.8 Medication effects

Medication effect	Examples
Vasodilation	Glycerol trinitrate, sodium nitroprusside
Vasoconstriction	Noradrenaline (norepinephrine), adrenaline (epinephrine), dopamine (above 5 mg/kg/min)
Increased cardiac contractility	Dopamine (below 5 mg/kg/min) dobutamine, isoprenaline
Anti-arrhythmia	Digoxin, amiodarone, adenosine
Antihypertensive	Atenolol, labetalol, nifedipine

THORACIC SURGERY

Types of Surgery

The following require a thoracotomy incision (see Appendix 2):

- **Pneumonectomy** = removal of whole lung.
- **Lobectomy** = removal of entire lobe (rest of lung will expand to fill space, hemidiaphragm will be slightly raised).
- **Sleeve resection** = section of bronchus removed ± lobectomy.
- **Segmentectomy** = excision of one or more of the bronchial segments.
- **Wedge resection** = removal of small localized tumour (usually non-malignant), or section of lung for biopsy.
- **Pleurectomy** = parietal pleura partially stripped, visceral pleura sticks to raw surface of chest wall.
- **Decortication** = thickened visceral pleura removed, allowing lung to re-expand and stick to parietal pleura. Rib resection is often required.
- **Lung volume reduction surgery** = removal of bullous areas of lung tissue.

- **Pleurodesis** = a chemical irritant + local anaesthetic inserted either through a chest drain or a thoroscope to set off an inflammatory response to adhere the two layers of pleura.
- **Lung transplant** is often performed through uni- or bilateral thoracotomy incision.
- **Thoracoplasty** is the removal of several ribs resulting in the collapse inwards of the chest wall. Very rarely used for unresolving empyema or for the surgical treatment of TB.
- **Oesophagectomy** is performed through a thoracotomy and a laparotomy, and two small cervical incisions.
- **Congenital deformities** e.g. pectus excavatum (funnel chest) and pectus carinatum (pigeon chest).
- **Repair of hiatus hernia** either through a left thoracotomy or a laparotomy.
- **Thorascopy** – used for investigations/biopsy.

Aims of Physiotherapy
- prevent sputum retention
- ensure inflation of remaining lung tissue
- ensure early mobility
- prevent shoulder/thoracic stiffness.

Table 14.9 Common problems in thoracic surgery

Common problems	Treatment modifications
Pain	• Analgesia MUST be optimized to allow effective cough • Usually use epidural or PCA • Note level and distribution of epidural. Check lower limb motor function • Fear of coughing – reassure, offer effective wound support
Delayed lung reinflation	• Chest drain on suction (pressure usually between −10 and 20 kPa) • Encourage mobility/use of exercise bike if appropriate
Sputum retention/chest infection	• Effective chest clearance essential. Discuss positive pressure treatments with surgeons • See Chapter 6
Air leak/surgical emphysema	• Air will escape through chest drain reducing efficacy of positive pressure techniques

table continues

Common problems	Treatment modifications
High surgical anastomosis	• Caution, if suction is agreed as essential – measure catheter from nose/mouth/tube to well above anastomosis, mark and suction with care
Reduced shoulder range of movement	• Ensure that patient is moving shoulder on operation side, especially flexion and abduction

Table 14.10 Common issues in thoracic surgery

Common issues	Advice
Patient knowledge of operation findings	• Diagnosis/outcome may not be discussed with a patient immediately – refer any questions to nurse/doctor looking after the patient
Pneumonectomy	• Side-lying with operation side uppermost is discouraged as remaining fluid in lung cavity may cause breakdown of anastomosis and leakage into lung (check your local policy) • Caution with suctioning as could damage anastomosis site, measure suction catheter if needed • Consent from surgical team for positive pressure techniques. Risk to anastomosis (usually tested to 40 mmHg in theatre) • Cavity fills gradually with fluid • If it fills too quickly the mediastinum will shift to unaffected lung side causing potential cardiac compromise • Discuss with the medical team if a shift is seen on CXR
Oesophagectomy	• Neck extension is avoided to prevent overstretching of anastomosis • Head down position should be avoided to prevent gastric reflux
Lung transplant	• Due to denervation patient may not cough spontaneously. Teach effective chest clearance • Gravity assisted positions may be of benefit • Care to be taken if suctioning due to anastomosis • Patients may be frail and malnourished preoperatively. This will limit exercise tolerance postoperatively • These patients often have postoperative complications and can deteriorate fast – assess and treat thoroughly
Chest drains (Fig. 14.1)	• Aim is to remove air and/or fluid from pleural space • Bottle to be kept below chest level • Bubbling shows air leak

	• If bubbling suddenly stops check for kink, blockage or disconnection of tube • Swinging is normal, showing changes in pleural pressure on breathing (if not on suction)
Empyema (infected pleural space)	• Usually presents a few weeks after surgery • Often treated by inserting a pigtail drain
Bronchopleural fistula	• Most common after pneumonectomy. Certain positions may need to be avoided to prevent any drainage into healthy lung

THORACIC SURGERY CALL OUT

Table 14.11 What do you need to ask?

Information source	What do you need to ask?
Telephone	• What operation? and has recovery been routine? • Is analgesia optimized, patient in good position, humidification? • Recent CXR?
From the ward staff	• Is the patient able to mobilize as part of treatment (if appropriate)? • If prescribed bronchodilators, have these been given?
From the charts/ monitors	• Observe chest drains
Key assessment points	• Check CXR • Check lower limb motor function if epidural being used • Ensure patient able to cough

Table 14.12 Treatment precautions

Treatment precautions	Explanation
Positive pressure techniques	• Check local policy; discuss with surgical team • If patient has large air leak consider how effective this would be
Positioning	• Check local policy for pneumonectomy and oesophagectomy patients
Suctioning	• If the suture line (anastomosis) is high, i.e. vulnerable to pressure from the suction catheter
Mobilizing	• If epidural is affecting patients lower limb motor function

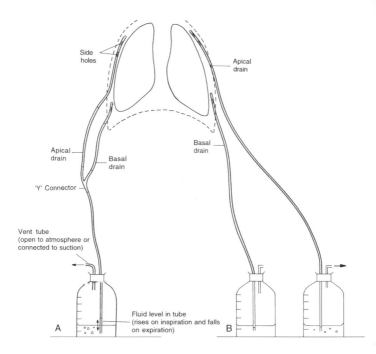

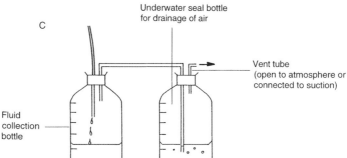

Figure 14.1 Underwater seal chest drainage. **A.** Single bottle system allowing use of one bottle via a 'Y' connector to drain fluid and air. **B.** Two separate bottles enabling drainage of air from the apical drain and fluid from the basal drain. **C.** Two compartment drainage system where two bottles are connected in series, the first collecting fluid and the second acting as the underwater seal drainage for air. Reproduced with kind permission from Pryor and Prasad (2002).

Table 14.13 Treatment contraindications

Treatment contraindications	Explanation
Positive pressure techniques	• Undrained pneumothorax

CHEST TRAUMA

• There are three main types of chest trauma: penetrating, crush or blunt injuries.

• Rupture of the diaphragm can occur due to an injury to the chest or abdomen following a RTA or as a result of a penetrating wound. There is a risk of an empyema as the stomach contents may leak into the pleural space.

• Very uncommon for trachea to be partially or totally disrupted. If wide separation patient usually will die.

• Sternal fractures are rare, and very painful. Ensure that the patient is assessed for cardiac damage.

Aims of Physiotherapy

• reduce work of breathing
• prevent sputum retention – humidification is essential
• minimize volume loss
• ensure early mobility.

Table 14.14 Common problems in chest trauma

Common problems	Treatment modifications
Pain	• Optimize analgesia; nerve blocks can be very useful; chest infection will follow injury unless patient can expectorate – especially if recent smoker or smoke inhalation
Lung contusions/ bleeding	• Ensure effective humidification (heated is ideal) • Blood in lung tissue becomes very difficult to expectorate; may cause $\downarrow$SpO$_2$ – heated, humidified CPAP can be very effective – try intermittent mouth piece/nose clip if mask inappropriate • Haemothorax will require a chest drain
Rib fractures	• Ensure no evidence of pneumo/haemothorax • Ensure adequate analgesia • If poor expansion consider IPPB/CPAP

table continues

Common problems	Treatment modifications
Flail chest (two or more ribs are fractured in more than one place)	• Chest movement is paradoxical (on inspiration the segment is sucked in and blown out on expiration) • CPAP to splint rib cage and stabilize movement and thus reduce pain
Pneumothorax	• Check drain observations and CXR

Table 14.15 Common issues in chest trauma

Common issues	Advice
Cardiac tamponade	• Check for signs ↑HR, ↑CVP, ↓BP
Hazard: other injuries	• Check notes carefully for all other injuries, e.g. facial, spinal, base of skull fractures

CARDIOTHORACIC TRAUMA CALL OUT

Table 14.16 What do you need to ask?

Information source	What do you need to ask?
Telephone	• Presenting problem? • Recent CXR? • Is analgesia optimal? • Can the patient be repositioned and effective humidification established?
From the ward staff	• Current status? • Establish when the patient may be busy/absent from the ward to avoid wasted time
From the charts/monitors	• CVS status?
Key assessment points	• Efficacy of pain control? • Ease of sputum clearance?

Table 14.17 Treatment precautions

Treatment precautions	Explanation
Manual techniques	• Will be very uncomfortable if have fractured ribs/flail chest

Table 14.18 Treatment contraindications

Treatment contraindications	Explanation
Positive pressure techniques	• Undrained pneumothorax

Key messages

- Empower the patient to undertake effective treatment.
- If possible all patients will benefit from early mobilization.
- Ensure patients have optimal analgesia.

References

Pryor JA, Prasad SA (eds) (2002) Physiotherapy for respiratory and cardiac problems, 3rd edn. London: Churchill Livingstone.

Further reading

Hinds CJ, Watson D (1996) Intensive care: a concise text book, 2nd edn. London: WB Saunders.
Singer M, Webb A (1997) Oxford handbook of critical care. Oxford: Oxford University Press.

CHAPTER 15 Calls to the oncology/ haematology unit

Katharine Malhotra and Nicola Thompson

The purpose of this chapter is to highlight different terminology and specific issues pertinent to the cancer patient:

- Cancer is treated by three main treatment modalities – surgery, radiotherapy and chemotherapy.
- Usually these are used in combination to provide the most effective treatment.
- Treatment depends on the site of the primary cancer, histology and the stage of disease on diagnosis.

As a physiotherapist you will need to be aware that many patients with cancer may have poor performance status prior to treatment. This may increase the risk of respiratory complications and impact upon their ability to comply with physiotherapy intervention.

This chapter covers patients presenting with respiratory compromise secondary to:

- bone marrow depression
- acute oncology
- metastatic oncology
- terminal phase of care.

BONE MARROW DEPRESSION

- side-effect of chemotherapy
- increases risk of infection, generally reverse barrier nursed
- more common with leukaemia, myeloma and lymphoma
- includes neutropenia, thrombocytopenia and anaemia.

Table 15.1 Common issues in bone marrow depression

Common issues	Advice
Neutropenia	• A low white cell count ($<0.5 \times 10^9$/L) • It is difficult to mount a normal response to infection, patient may present with an unproductive cough and ↑work of breathing • Use positioning to assist breathing control
Hazard: thrombocytopenia	• A low platelet count ($<150 \times 10^9$/L) • Commonest cause of bleeding in haemato-oncological conditions • Platelets prevent bleeding • Patients who are febrile or septic do not maintain platelet levels and require extra support with platelet transfusion • All hospitals should have a policy for when to transfuse • Generally, platelets are transfused when levels have dropped between 10 and 20×10^9/L • Physiotherapy intervention should take place during or immediately after platelet transfusion • Need to know count • Need to know if actively bleeding • Minimize intervention if actively bleeding, i.e. positioning and breathing exercises • If requiring suction, ensure count above 20×10^9/L (check local policy/seek medical advice) • Can suction while platelets being transfused • Manual techniques, i.e. percussion and vibrations, can be used. Use a towel to decrease risk of bruising
Anaemia	• A low haemoglobin (Hb) count **[<13.5 g/dL in men and <11.5 g/dL in women]** • Anaemia occurs in haemato-oncological malignancies due to ↓red cell production and primary disease process itself • Most centres attempt to keep a patient's Hb level >8 g/dL • Patients may present with shortness of breath on exertion (SOBOE). Blood is unable to carry sufficient oxygen to the body's muscles therefore increasing the work of breathing • Physiotherapy is not appropriate; medical management should reverse symptoms

ACUTE ONCOLOGY

Table 15.2 Common issues in acute oncology

Common issues	Advice
Tumour occluding airway	• Primary lung cancer may cause airway obstruction, atelectasis $\pm$ consolidation behind the tumour, and inflammation around the tumour • Patient may present with stridor, a harsh wheeze requiring medical intervention • Patient may sound productive • Physiotherapy is not appropriate to clear secretions from behind a tumour that fully occludes airway • Ensure good positioning to ↓work of breathing, O_2 therapy, adequate analgesia and monitor • Physiotherapy may be appropriate after primary therapy has shrunk tumour or if tumour is partially occluding airway • Ensure adequate time for postural drainage techniques in this case
Hazard	• IPPB can be used but is CONTRAINDICATED with proximal tumours because of air trapping
Mucositis	• Inflammation of mucosa of mouth and throat is common after chemotherapy $\pm$ radiotherapy • Excessive production of thick, mucoid upper respiratory tract secretions with mouth soreness and ulceration are common • Patients find it difficult to clear secretions • Mucositis may be mistaken for chest infection • Advice on breathing exercises and use of high volume lung clearance techniques to clear upper airway • Regular saline nebulizers may enable easier passage of secretions • Chest infection may coexist – look for specific chest signs
Aspergillosis	• Opportunistic fungal infection • Occurs with prolonged neutropenia and with severe bone marrow depression

	• Bronchopulmonary aspergilloma can cause cavitating lesions and invade small blood vessels • Symptoms include malaise, weight loss, fever and productive cough $\pm$ haemoptysis • If infective sputum present use manual techniques/positioning/adequate humidification for mucous plugging • No physiotherapy if frank haemoptysis
Pneumocystis carinii pneumonia (PCP)	• Opportunistic infection in immunocompromised patients causing inflammation of the lungs • Organisms damage the alveolar lining and produce a foamy exudate • Symptoms include a dry cough, $\uparrow$respiratory rate, breathlessness, hypoxaemia and fever • Auscultation may often reveal fine, diffuse crackles • X-ray appearances usually show a bilateral haze in the hilar region developing into diffuse symmetrical shadowing (butterfly) • Medical treatment is with O_2 therapy, respiratory support (CPAP or NIV) and antibiotics • Physiotherapy advice on positioning for relaxation, breathing control and mobilization may be beneficial
Pneumonitis	• Inflammatory condition which may be progressive • Radiation-induced, drug-related or of viral origin, e.g. cytomegalovirus (CMV) • Patients present with a dry cough, $\uparrow$respiratory rate and breathlessness • Medical treatment is with high dose steroids in acute stages • Physiotherapy advice on positioning for relaxation and breathing control may be beneficial
Disseminated intravascular coagulation (DIC)	• A bleeding disorder with an alteration in the blood clotting mechanism • Caused by an underlying disease process and is always a secondary condition

table continues

Common issues	Advice
	• Major causes in the haemato-oncology population are severe sepsis and acute promyelocytic leukaemia
	• Advise caution with physiotherapy intervention due to risk of haemorrhage, therefore no manual techniques/IPPB/PEP
Pulmonary embolus	• Obstruction to the pulmonary artery or branches by a thrombus
	• Symptoms include breathlessness of sudden onset, pleuritic chest pain, $\downarrow SpO_2$ and haemoptysis
	• Increased risk with compression or invasion of pulmonary system, DIC and non-ambulatory patient
	• Physiotherapy is not appropriate – medical management with anticoagulation and O_2 therapy

METASTATIC ONCOLOGY

Table 15.3 Common issues in metastatic oncology

Common issues	Advice
Hazard: spinal cord compression	• Caused by primary or metastatic cancer by extradural or intradural compression on spinal cord
	• **An oncological emergency → primary treatment with surgery, radiotherapy or occasionally chemotherapy is vital to minimize neurological deterioration**
	• May occur at any spinal level and is characterized by motor and sensory loss below level of impairment with bladder and bowel changes
	• Patients may experience respiratory difficulties depending on level of compression. Abdominal muscles may also be compromised reducing the patient's ability to cough
	• Physiotherapy options will depend on stability of spine, condition of patient and adequate pain control
	• **Check with medics re: stability of spine prior to physiotherapy (refer to Ch. 13)**

	• Intervention can include positioning, ACBT, assisted cough and use of IPPB to assist with sputum clearance and ability to cough
Hazard: bony metastatic disease	• Often associated with pain and can lead to pathological fracture and hypercalcaemia
	• Common in breast cancer, prostate cancer, lung cancer and myeloma patients
	• Usually affects long bones or flat bones of skeleton
	• Important to check for presence of bony disease prior to chest physiotherapy via X-rays/scan reports if available
	• Adequate analgesia needs to be considered prior to treatment to ensure appropriate positioning
	• Use positive pressure adjuncts
	• One-handed percussion may be used if necessary, using a towel for cushioning
Caution – rib fracture may occur	• Use chest vibrations even if rib metastases are present if no other technique is successful and sputum clearance is important. If unsure discuss risk/benefit to patient with team – report immediately if occurs to ensure pain relief
	• ↓Risk by ensuring patient feedback for comfort/pain
Hypercalcaemia	• ↑Serum calcium levels usually associated with presence of bony metastatic disease
	• Symptoms include confusion, lethargy, nausea and vomiting, constipation and thirst
	• Physiotherapists need to be aware of this condition as symptoms may compromise effective treatment
Pleural effusion	• Excessive amount of fluid in pleural space
	• Symptoms include pallor, cyanosis, dyspnoea, ↑respiratory rate, ↓breath sounds and dullness to percussion on the affected side, ↓peripheral O_2 saturations and chest pain
	• Pleural effusion can be readily identified on CXR
	• Causes pressure upon the surrounding lung tissue
	• Medical treatment is by insertion of intrapleural drain
	• Physiotherapy is not appropriate in acute call out situation
Superior vena cava obstruction (SVCO)	• Primary or metastatic in nature
	• Caused by extrinsic or intrinsic compression of superior vena cava

table continues

Common issues	Advice
	• Usually associated with lung cancer with direct compression from a mass in the right main bronchus or lymphoma with compression from the mediastinal or paratracheal lymph nodes • Presents with swelling of neck, upper trunk, upper extremity, dyspnoea with hypoxia, cough and chest pain • Medical treatment is essential with radiotherapy or chemotherapy • Physiotherapy is not appropriate
Ascites	• Excessive fluid in peritoneal cavity • Symptoms include abdominal distension and discomfort, nausea and vomiting, leg oedema, and dyspnoea • Medical treatment is with drug therapy and drainage of peritoneal cavity via a catheter (paracentesis) • Ascites will compromise diaphragmatic excursion • Positioning will be difficult • Forward lean sitting/side-lying may be options
Lymphangitis carcinomatosa	• Diffuse infiltration of lymphatics of lungs by cancer cells • Symptoms include dyspnoea, cough $\pm$ pleuritic chest pain and central cyanosis • Medical treatment is with drug therapy (corticosteroids and O_2 therapy) • Physiotherapy is not appropriate • Advice on positioning may be of some benefit to assist breathing control

TERMINAL STAGE OF DISEASE

Table 15.4 Common issues in terminal disease

Common issues	Advice
Death rattle	• A rattling noise produced by secretions oscillating in time with inspiration and expiration • Can be distressing for relatives, carers and other patients • Antisecretory agents are useful, e.g. glycopyrronium or hyoscine. Physiotherapy is not appropriate but

	explanation that patient is not distressed may ease families' anxieties
	• Advice regarding positioning may be beneficial
	• Would not encourage use of suction as can increase secretions further
	• If patient distressed advice on regular suction may be appropriate. This does not have to be a physiotherapy intervention
Terminal restlessness	• Common in period immediately preceding death
	• Use of sedation may be necessary to keep patient comfortable

Remember:
- Physiotherapy intervention is limited in these stages.
- It can be distressing to feel helpless in these situations but you should feel able to recognize your professional limitations.
- Support should be sought from peers.

Table 15.5 Specific equipment

Specific equipment	Notes for physiotherapists
Hickman catheter	• Used for long-term venous access
	• Skin-tunnelled catheter lying in subcutaneous tunnel and exiting midway from anterior chest wall
	• Introduced via subclavian vein
	• Tip lies in superior vena cava or right atrium
Syringe driver	• Portable battery operated infusion pump
	• Used for administration of drugs via a subcutaneous route
	• Used for analgesics, antiemetics, dexamethasone and anxiolytic sedatives
	• Often inserted into upper arm or thigh
Epidural infusion via an in-dwelling spinal catheter	• Epidural analgesia is administration of analgesics into epidural space
	• Used for postoperative pain control or treatment of chronic intractable pain

KEY POINTS FOR THE CALL OUT

Solid Tumours

From the Referrer
- Sudden/gradual change in condition?
- Where is the cancer?
- Stage of treatment, i.e. acute/palliative?
- Other chest disease, i.e. pleural effusion, circulatory complications?
- Productive cough?

From the Notes, X-Rays and Scan Results
- Bony metastatic spread?
- Site of infection in relation to tumour?
- White cell count?
- Resuscitation status?
- Check for pleural effusion.

Table 15.6 Common problems

Common problems	Treatment precautions/modifications
• Fatigue	• Shorten treatment time
• Bony metastatic disease, rib disease	• Risk of rib fracture with manual techniques
	• Feedback from patient essential re: comfort/pain
	• Balance necessity for treatment against risks
• Spinal cord compression	• Check the stability of spine prior to treatment
• Pain	• Modify positions
	• Consider analgesia
• Tumour occluding airway	• Physiotherapy will not clear secretions from behind a tumour
• Terminal phase of disease	• Think about patient comfort – you may not change the pathology

Haematological Malignancies

From the Referrer
- Sudden/gradual change in condition?
- ↑Temperature?
- White cell/platelet counts? If transfusion planned, when for?
- Productive cough?
- Are respiratory difficulties related to inflammatory changes?

From the Notes, X-Rays and Scan Results
- Bony metastatic spread (myeloma)?
- Blood counts?
- Resuscitation status?
- Recent cancer treatment?

Table 15.7 Common problems

Common problems	Treatment precautions/modifications
• WOB	• Position to assist breathing control • Reassurance • Do not rush
• Sputum retention	• Low platelet count therefore care with all techniques • Ensure not due to tumour obstruction
• Fatigue	• Shorten treatment time
• Unproductive cough	• Position to assist breathing control • Reassurance ± relaxation • Medical advice re: simple linctus (cough suppressant)/lidocaine (lignocaine)
• Bony metastatic disease, rib disease	• Risk of rib fracture with manual techniques • Feedback from patient essential re: comfort/pain • Balance necessity for treatment against risks

Further reading

Grundy M (ed) (2000) Nursing in haematological oncology. London: Baillière Tindall.

Hoffbrand AV, Pettit JE (1999) Essential haematology, 3rd edn. Oxford: Blackwell Science.

Hough A (2001) Physiotherapy in respiratory care, 3rd edn. Cheltenham: Stanley Thornes.

Mallet J, Dougherty L (2000) The Royal Marsden Hospital manual of clinical nursing procedures, 5th edn. Oxford: Blackwell Science.

Otto SE (ed) (1997) Oncology nursing, 3rd edn. St Louis: Mosby.

Thompson N, Chittenden T (1998) The sepsis syndrome and the cancer patient: respiratory management and active physiotherapy. Eur J Cancer Care 7:99–101.

Tschudin V (1996) Nursing the patient with cancer, 2nd edn. London: Prentice Hall.

Twycross R, Wilcock A (2001) Symptom management in advanced cancer, 3rd edn. Oxford: Radcliffe Medical Press.

CHAPTER
16

Calls to the paediatric unit

Paul Ritson

It is sometimes more daunting to be called to a paediatric ward than it is to be called to the paediatric intensive care unit (PICU). The levels of monitoring on the wards are much less than you would find on a PICU, so your observational skills will be vitally important. From the moment the telephone rings to the time you start treatment, you must constantly gather appropriate information, analyse it and formulate a plan of action.

INAPPROPRIATE CALLS

Unfortunately, your call out may sometimes be inappropriate. Table 16.1 lists some conditions that require extreme caution when treating or are totally contraindicated for treatment.

Table 16.1 Conditions requiring caution and contraindications

Condition	Explanation
Stridor	• **Do not touch!** • Harsh sound heard on inspiration • Caused by swelling/oedema/obstruction in upper airway • Usual treatment includes humidification, adrenaline (epinephrine), nebulizers or intubation/tracheostomy
Croup	• Viral inflammation of upper respiratory tract • Barking cough • Do not touch unless airway protected by endotracheal tube
Bronchiolitis	• Inflammation of bronchioles • Usually in winter

	• Physiotherapy will cause hypoxia • Treat only superimposed chest infection/lobar collapse
Whooping cough (pertussis)	• Upper respiratory tract swelling • Paroxysmal cough and vomiting • Physiotherapy may make patient worse • Apnoeas common • May require ventilation
Acute epiglottitis	• Swollen epiglottis • **Do not touch!** • Airway blocks off quickly • Child should be sat upright with head/neck extended
Acute pneumonia	• Consolidation phase • Non-productive and painful
Bronchospasm	• Treat cause of bronchospasm prior to attempting treatment
Inhaled foreign bodies	• Common in children/toddlers • Do not be persuaded to treat! • Bronchoscopic removal first, then physiotherapy if indicated
Undrained pneumothorax	• Do not use IPPB/CPAP • Could cause tension pneumothorax • Position for ventilation/perfusion until chest drain inserted
Severe CVS instability	• Physiotherapy contraindicated • Use of IPPB/CPAP contraindicated
Severe raised ICP	• Physiotherapy can increase ICP
Uncontrolled seizures	• Hypoxia and aspiration may occur during seizures – assess when seizure activity reduces
Pulmonary embolus/ clotting disorders	• Patient may bleed or throw off clots if treated

KEY ASSESSMENT NOTES

When assessing a paediatric patient, it is vitally important to assess all of the body's systems as they all interact and can affect your assessment and treatment of choice.

Cardiovascular System

Is the patient cardiovascularly stable?

Table 16.2   Assessment of cardiovascular stability

Blood pressure	• Is BP normal for child's age? (see Ch. 4 for normal values)
Heart rate	• Is the heart rate normal for the child's age?
	• Is the heart rhythm normal sinus rhythm?

Neurological System

Could the patient's neurological status affect your treatment?

Table 16.3   Assessment of neurological status

Temperature	• Infants can suffer seizures if pyrexial (febrile convulsion)
Intracranial pressure (ICP)	• Head injured patients should be monitored closely for abnormal neurological signs
Pre-existing pathology	• Does the patient have a neurological condition that causes respiratory problems or alters your treatment choice, e.g. Duchenne muscular dystrophy

Orthopaedic

Does your patient have any orthopaedic problems that could affect your treatment?

Table 16.4   Assessment of orthopaedic problems

Fractures	• Spinal and limb fractures will affect the positioning of your patient
	• Follow your hospital's protocols carefully
Pre-existing conditions	• Kyphoscoliosis, chest or limb deformities alter the normal mechanics of respiration, predisposing to respiratory disease
	• Positioning will also be difficult, but still try to position effectively
Surgery	• Orthopaedic surgery, especially spinal, can change the mechanics of respiration and will dictate the positions your patient is allowed to be in
	• Follow your hospital's protocols carefully

Fluid Balance

Table 16.5 Fluid balance assessment

| Positive balance | • Expect copious loose secretions and pulmonary oedema |
| Negative balance | • Thick viscous secretions leading to mucous plugging and sputum retention |

Drugs

Review the patient's drug charts.

Table 16.6 Review of drug chart

Inotropes	• Cardiovascular support drugs, usually only seen on PICU • E.g. adrenaline (epinephrine), dobutamine, enoximone, noradrenaline (norepinephrine), dopamine
Painkillers	• Look at the route of administration, i.v., i.m., oral, rectal, epidural • E.g. morphine, Voltarol, paracetamol, fentanyl • Is pain relief adequate? Does it require time to take effect?
Sedatives	• Look at route of administration • E.g. midazolam, Phenergan, chloral hydrate, clonidine (propofol not used in children under 1 year)
Bronchodilators	• Must be given before physiotherapy and before inhaled steroids • In infants, current research suggests B2 agonists are effective; however, some controversy still exists • Salbutamol and ipratropium bromide can both be used as a treatment for bronchospasm • E.g. ipratropium bromide (Atrovent), salbutamol (Ventolin), terbutaline sulphate (Bricanyl)
Steroids	• Inhaled or systemic • E.g. prednisolone, budesonide (Pulmicort) • Long-term systemic steroids cause osteoporosis, even in children
Diuretics	• Could indicate pre-existing cardiac pathology or pulmonary oedema • E.g. furosemide (frusemide), captopril

Carry out a full paediatric respiratory assessment, including type of surgery, incision site, relevant past history and special postoperative instructions.

AIMS OF PHYSIOTHERAPY TREATMENT

- prevent/treat atelectasis
- aid removal of secretions
- reduce work of breathing (WOB)
- ensure adequate analgesia
- gain patient/parent trust and cooperation.

CALLS TO THE PAEDIATRIC SURGICAL WARD

Table 16.7 Common problems in the paediatric surgical ward

Common problems	Treatment modifications
Atelectasis	• Good positioning is essential • Sitting upright is effective for infants who frequently suffer upper lobe collapse – use a car seat to achieve this, making sure the patient is safe and supported • Alternate side-lying aids re-expansion of uppermost lung; regular repositioning is essential • Blowing games or bubble bottles and incentive spirometers are useful in older children • If able, mobilize patient. This may involve play, standing at a table to play or other creative ways of encouraging children to their feet! • IPPB and CPAP can be used effectively. It is suggested that most children aged 6 years and over are able to comply with IPPB
Sputum retention	• Occurs due to pain, immobility or inability to cough for whatever reason • Ensure adequate analgesia • Humidify with face mask in children and head box in infants • 5 ml 0.9% saline nebulizers can be used hourly • If patient unable to cough spontaneously or to command, oropharyngeal or nasopharyngeal suction may be indicated if secretions adversely affecting patient • Position for comfort and drainage • Assess use of 'head down' – tip very carefully as reflux, vomiting and aspiration occur more easily

	in this position. This has a detrimental impact upon diaphragmatic function in babies, especially after abdominal surgery • Mobilize patient if possible • Use teddies or dolls for wound support when coughing
Increased work of breathing	• 'Head up' position reduces load on diaphragm and reduces reflux of gastric contents • Avoid supine as worst position for gas exchange and increases risk of aspiration during vomiting • Alternate side-lying with head up reduces load on diaphragm and improves gas exchange • Prone lying best position for gas exchange and reducing WOB – not commonly used on spontaneously breathing patients because of link to sudden infant death syndrome (cot death)
	• **If using prone lying, patient MUST be closely monitored** by nursing staff and have the following monitors in situ: SpO_2, apnoea mat, ECG, all with alarms enabled and audible

Table 16.8   Common issues in the paediatric surgical ward

Common issues	Advice
Pain	• An infant in pain usually cries inconsolably • A child in pain will also cry but can also be unusually quiet until disturbed • A child in pain will not be cooperative! • Check timing of analgesia and route of administration – how long will it take to become effective? • Can supplemental analgesia be given? Beware of opiate depression of the CNS • Cooperative children can use Entonox if prescribed and the clinician is trained to administer • Entonox can be used in infants but must be carefully assessed and used as above
Poor cooperation	• A common problem! • See Chapter 3 • Try trickery, use toys or play, i.e. incentive spirometer, blow bottle, bubbles • Distraction by parents/nurses during treatment

table continues

Common issues	Advice
	• **Never** force or hold down unless the child is in danger
Poor position	• Child in pain is usually slumped in bed in a flexed position – use supported positioning to improve pain and respiratory function • Children/infants with neurological disorders can have increased extensor tone when in pain – ensure adequate pain relief and optimize position • Early mobilization/sit out of bed if possible
Parents	• See Chapter 3 • Will be very anxious • Always gain consent for treatment • Gain parents' trust and cooperation • Involve parents in treatment if possible • Children may be more cooperative if parents are not around at time of treatment • Some children may only do treatment with parent
Oxygen delivery	• Humidification is vital if secretions are thick or if oxygen%/FiO_2 >28%/0.28 • Use head box or face mask – never nasal cannulae – for humidification
Timing of treatment	• Never treat a patient after a feed or meal because of the risk of vomiting/aspiration • Leave at least 1 h before treating • Preferably, treat prior to a feed/meal
Blocked nose	• Can cause increased work of breathing even in the absence of other pathologies • Unblock nose if possible • Saline drops can be used to moisten crusted nasal secretions
Other pathologies	• Be aware of the patient with complex multiple needs on the surgical ward – it is this type of patient that deteriorates very quickly

COMMON CONDITIONS SEEN ON PAEDIATRIC SURGICAL WARDS

There are many conditions encountered on the surgical wards. All conditions should be taken into consideration when carrying out a respiratory assessment. Further reading about conditions is strongly recommended.

Table 16.9 Assessment/treatment advice for common conditions on paediatric surgical wards

Condition	Assessment/treatment hints
Idiopathic kyphoscoliosis (postoperative correction)	• Altered respiratory mechanics postoperatively • Chest drains for at least 1 week • Ribs removed during surgery, care with manual techniques • Must log roll to side-lie – no rotation allowed • Incentive spirometry very effective
Cerebral palsy (CP)	• Usually postop orthopaedic surgery in hip spica • General surgery for fundoplication and/or gastrostomy • Pain and sputum retention usually main problems exacerbated by poor cough • Positioning is vital for respiratory and neurological reasons
Congenital cardiac disorders: • Atrial septal defect (ASD) • Ventricular septal defect (VSD) • Tetralogy of Fallot (TOF) • Atrioventricular septal defect (AVSD) • Transposition of great arteries (TGA) (to name a few)	• Full paediatric respiratory assessment • Take special note of patient's colour and SpO_2 – cyanosis is common and normal in many cardiac conditions: • Fallot's tetralogy pre-repair >80% • Blalock–Taussig shunts >80% • Central shunts >80% • Fenestrated Fontan >80% • Complete Fontan repair >90% • Damus–Kaye >70% • Cavopulmonary anastomosis >80% • Rastelli repair >95% • TGA pre-septostomy >50–70% • TGA post-septostomy >80% • Switch repair of TGA >95% • Pulmonary stenosis (PS) pre-ballooning >70% • PS post-ballooning >85% • VSD >95% • VSD with pulmonary artery band >70%
	• Above to be used as a guide only – each child may have slightly different accepted SpO_2 limits

table continues

Condition	Assessment/treatment hints
Congenital diaphragmatic hernia repair	• Depending on size and duration of hernia, diaphragm may be weakened and affected lung may be underdeveloped/hypoplastic, predisposing to respiratory insufficiency
Abdominal surgery	• Can cause distension, leading to splinting of diaphragm – use high side-lying to aid diaphragm excursion

Table 16.10 Monitors and equipment

Monitors and equipment	Explanation
Patient controlled analgesia (PCA) or nurse controlled analgesia (NCA)	• If old enough, the child will be able to press for pain relief • If younger or passive patient, the nurse **ONLY** can press button for pain relief
Pulse oximeter	• Very commonly used postoperatively • Make sure the probe is attached to patient and signal is strong • Look at the patient as well as the oximeter – if the SpO_2 says 30% and patient is pink the oximeter is likely to be wrong!
Chest drains	• Never clamp unless lifting drain above waist level

CALLS TO THE PAEDIATRIC MEDICAL WARD

Carry out a full paediatric respiratory assessment, including past history and the course of this episode. In this group of patients, pre-existing pathology may be particularly relevant.

Table 16.11 Common problems on the paediatric medical ward

Common problems	Treatment modifications
Atelectasis (as surgical patient)	• Effective positioning is vital – always position the affected side uppermost to improve ventilation and sputum clearance. If the patient desaturates, the dependent lung may be too squashed – try modifying the position

	• Position affected side down to improve oxygenation if hypoxic
	• Avoid 'head down' position in infants/children with history of aspiration and/or reflux
	• IPPB/CPAP useful – be careful with IPPB or CPAP pressures
	• Mobilize patient if possible
Sputum retention (as surgical patient)	• Occurs commonly in children with neurological disorders, e.g. CP, spina bifida (SB), muscular dystrophy, spinal muscular atrophy (SMA)
	• Due to poor cough, altered mechanics of respiration or aspiration
	• Oropharyngeal (OP) or nasopharyngeal (NP) suction can be very important in this group of patients. The technique is sometimes tricky – other staff may be able to assist
	• Care with OP suction as this can stimulate the gag reflex and induce vomiting
	• Positioning in alternate side-lying with head up is effective for sputum removal and comfort
	• Ensure adequate humidification via face mask, or head box
	• Humidification is essential if $FiO_2 > 0.28$
	• 5 ml 0.9% NaCl nebulizers can be given hourly if secretions viscous – must be prescribed
	• Tracheal rub may be useful if cough is poor and it is accepted unit policy
	• Some patients may have used a cough assist machine at home or on a previous admission – only use if you or the nursing staff are familiar with it. See Chapter 18
Increased work of breathing (as surgical patient)	• Ascertain cause of increased WOB and treat accordingly
	• Position is the most important treatment
	• High side-lying, supported sitting are useful
	• Treat in quiet area if possible
	• Ensure nappy or clothes are not too tight – compressing abdomen can increase WOB

Common Issues on the Paediatric Medical Ward

Many of the issues encountered on the medical ward are similar to those seen on the surgical ward. Those more commonly encountered on the medical ward are mentioned in Table 16.12.

Table 16.12 Common issues and advice

Common issues	Advice
Poor position	• Good positioning is essential for effective respiration • Avoid supine, unless being used as a specific drainage position
Inappropriate oxygen delivery	• Beware the dangers of high flow dry oxygen! • Always humidify • Don't try to humidify via nasal cannulae
Bronchospasm	• Ascertain cause • Bronchodilator 30 min prior to treatment and reassess • Given via nebulizer or spacer • Salbutamol is sometimes ineffective in infants but current research suggests that this may not be the case – discuss with the referring doctor • Small amounts of bronchodilator can be diluted with 0.9% NaCl • Salbutamol and ipratropium bromide can be mixed and given together
Uncooperative child	• Use play and distraction • Trickery! • Enlist parents' help or ask parents to leave if child 'acting up' with them around • Never force a child
Child with complex needs	• This type of patient may be unable to cooperate with treatment • Treatment usually passive • Speak to, and reassure patient • Don't attempt to lift/move a larger child by yourself – ask parents or nursing staff to help

Common Conditions Seen on the Paediatric Medical Ward

There are many conditions encountered on the medical wards. Pathologies behind these conditions must be taken into consideration when assessing these children. Further reading about conditions is strongly recommended.

Table 16.13 Common conditions and treatment advice

Condition	Assessment/treatment hints
Cystic fibrosis (CF)	• Will have set routine at home – check notes/ask parents pre-treatment so that you feel confident (see postural drainage positions/ACBT/PEP – Ch. 18). You may need to concentrate on certain positions • May have routine bronchodilator pre-treatment • DNase is given after treatment to liquefy sticky mucus – usually overnight • Check abdomen (soft or hard?) – will affect work of breathing if hard; discuss with team • Look at lung function tests and compare to previous tests • Exercise very important • Children often uncooperative • Be assertive (but not bossy!) • Never force or restrain a child unless they are in danger • Auscultation often deceptive – crackles sometimes not heard even in the presence of retained secretions • Listen to cough – does it sound dry, tight, productive, etc.? • Obtain sputum sample for culture and sensitivity if requested • NIV is sometimes used in older CF patients as a bridge to transplant or to aid respiratory function during acute episodes. NIV can be used overnight or continuously in certain circumstances. Always discuss with the nursing staff/referring doctor before removing the NIV mask/nasal pillows. Sputum clearance techniques can be used while the patient is on NIV and the mask removed only for expectoration if the patient is severely compromised
Asthma	• Positioning in acute phase • Use heated humidification if requiring oxygen • Ensure bronchospasm under control

table continues

Condition	Assessment/treatment hints
	• Beware of quiet lung sounds (overwhelming bronchospasm), fatigue and increasing CO_2 on ABGs – will need anaesthetic review
Bronchopulmonary dysplasia	• Many have home oxygen – find out normal FiO_2 • Tendency for bronchospasm • Treat as chronic lung disease
Primary ciliary dyskinesia	• Rare • Develop sputum retention/chest infection quickly
Immunodeficiency	• Treat chest symptoms as for CF
Neurological conditions: • Cerebral palsy (CP) • Spinal muscular atrophy (SMA) • Duchenne muscular dystrophy (DMD) • Congenital muscular dystrophy (CMD) • Spina bifida (SB)	• Aspiration, poor cough and sputum retention common • Ask parent (or child, if able) what chest is like normally – what you see may be normal for that child • Assisted cough using abdominal support is effective with degenerative disorders such as DMD/SMA • Gravity assisted positions used with care (risk of reflux/aspiration) • Use IPPB/CPAP and cough assist if indicated • OP/NP suction only if secretions are causing respiratory distress or patient is uncomfortable • Always talk to child • Get help to turn or position child • If repeated suction is necessary, or the patient is not protecting airway properly, use a nasopharyngeal airway • **NEVER** use an oropharyngeal airway (Geudel) in a conscious patient – risk of vomiting/aspiration
The dying child	• Very uncommon to be called out in these circumstances • Ascertain why the call out is being made and what the referrer expects Management for this group of patients may include: • Positioning to keep the child comfortable – side-lying or long sitting well supported with pillows

- Suction **only** if the patient is **distressed with secretions** and unable to expectorate – technique should be quick, gentle and effective
- Don't forget to talk to the child and the parents/carers
- Ensure that the child's dignity is maintained
- Remember that this is a distressing time for all concerned and that senior staff will always be available for help, advice and support
- Discuss with team the need for physiotherapy versus time with family, etc.
- Always check resuscitation status of child – is the child for no resuscitation, oxygen and suction only or for full resuscitation?

Key messages

- Be methodical.
- Gather appropriate information.
- Consider pre-existing pathologies.
- Communicate with the child, the parents and the multidisciplinary team.
- Never underestimate the power of play.
- Be very observant.
- Frequently reassess your patient.
- Be aware of signs of respiratory distress (Ch. 3) and contraindications/cautions.

Further reading

Jordan SC, Scott O (1989) Heart disease in paediatrics, 3rd edn. London: Butterworths.

Prasad SA, Hussey J (1995) Paediatric respiratory care: a guide for physiotherapists and health professionals. London: Chapman Hall.

Pryor JA, Prasad SA (2002) Physiotherapy for respiratory and cardiac problems, 3rd edn. Edinburgh: Churchill Livingstone.

Calls to the neonatal unit

Allie Carter

TO TREAT OR NOT TO TREAT?

Calls to the neonatal unit are rare now that a balance has been achieved between minimal handling and appropriate, timely repositioning of preterm babies to prevent secretion retention and lobar collapse.

The evidence base for treating this group of infants is lacking and therefore treatments should not be routine, but restricted to babies who display respiratory distress through specific lobar collapse or thick tenacious secretions.

> **Remember:**
> It is generally accepted that the treatment of this client group should not be undertaken unless the physiotherapist is fully trained in the care of neonates. If in doubt do not attempt to treat.

Often simple instructions regarding position changes and adequate suctioning are sufficient in an unstable baby. A deteriorating respiratory status as a result of lobar collapse or retention of secretions will indicate the need for more active assessment and intervention.

- **Neonate** = a baby born from 37 weeks (term is 40 weeks).
- **Premature baby** = a baby born before 37 weeks.

REASONS FOR RISK IN TREATING THESE INFANTS

- Extreme prematurity and low birth weight therefore a high incidence of instability with handling.
- Immature CNS and lungs.
- Long periods of time needed to recover after minimal interventions.

- High risk of secondary sequelae (e.g. cerebral bleeds, abdominal bleeds).

AIM OF PHYSIOTHERAPY

- To maintain/improve gaseous exchange without further compromising the already fragile, immature infant.

AIMS OF TREATMENT

- To maintain a clear airway.
- To assist in the removal of tenacious secretions.
- To improve gaseous exchange.
- To assist early extubation.
- To help prevent further respiratory collapse.

NORMAL VALUES

Table 17.1 Normal values

Normal values – brief outline	
Heart rate	• **[Preterm 100–200 b.p.m.]** • **[Term 80–200 b.p.m.]**
Blood pressure	• **[Approx. 80/45 mmHg]** • Aim to keep systolic above 35–45 mmHg
Respiratory rate	• **[Approx. 30–45 breaths per minute]**
Saturations	• **[90–96%]**

EQUIPMENT

- Ventilators vary between units. Nursing staff should be able to guide you.
- Ventilators with flow loops indicate the need for suction when the loop is interrupted by obstruction.
- CPAP units with nasal prongs or masks have led to infants being extubated earlier.
- Care is needed to keep the nasal passages patent.

COMMON PROBLEMS, CONDITIONS AND ISSUES

Table 17.2 Common problems in the neonatal unit

Common problems	Treatment modifications
Lobar collapse (frequently R upper lobe due to endotracheal tube being too long)	• Modify positioning • Ensure regular change of position to prevent further collapse • May use half lying/semi-propped position • Suction with head to the left • Record and discuss with nursing staff
Secretion retention Increased viscosity and amount	• Check humidification is adequate • Use of saline with treatment (see below) • Assess for evidence of infection and/or pulmonary oedema • Increase frequency of position change • May need increased frequency of suctioning especially if the infant has been turned 8 hourly

Table 17.3 Common conditions in neonates and term babies

Common conditions in neonates	
Respiratory distress syndrome With increased secretions and/or acute lobar collapse	• Regular change of position • Active techniques not indicated unless collapse is present which does not improve with repositioning and suction
Chronic lung disease With multifocal collapse Chronic secretion retention CO_2 retention	• Treatment as indicated • Regular change of position • Active techniques with effective suction • Daily assessment
Term baby – common problems Hypoxic ischaemic Encephalopathy Meconium aspiration Tracheo-oesophageal fistula Diaphragmatic hernia	• Limitations to positioning due to stability/operation site • Maintain frequency of position change • Effective suctioning • Treat collapse as required

| Cardiac anomalies term and preterm | • Treat only if indicated
• Attempt position change even if only minimal movement is possible
• Discuss the individual precautions of individual cardiac anomalies with medical and nursing staff |

Table 17.4 Common issues in the neonatal unit

Common issues	Advice
Routine treatments being undertaken	• Individual treatment plans are essential • Assess and reassess as constantly changing
Chest sounding clear but on assessment yield of copious secretions	• Often clinically indicated to clear secretions from the posterior lung bases • Place prone at least once in a 24-h period • Record/discuss with colleagues
Infants 28–29 weeks and under not tolerating side-lying	• Use quarter turns from prone and supine • Lungs not fully developed laterally • Rib cage very compliant • Quarter turns are tolerated better
Preferential ventilation	• In the presence of one-sided collapse the infant may not tolerate lying on the fully expanded lung, due to VQ mismatch • May need to increase the oxygen • Position change for drainage may only be possible for short periods of time • NB: Collapse on the opposite side may occur if an infant is nursed for long periods in one position • Record and set a plan

table continues

Common issues	Advice
Rapid desaturation with appropriate treatment/handling	• Can be pre-empted by pre-oxygenation • 15–20% initially • Use of manual breaths on ventilator if secondary bradycardia
Apnoeas of prematurity	• Common – may happen during treatment • Stimulate baby to breathe, tap bottom, flick heel • In emergency give manual breaths with a bag
Nursing position maintained for long periods of time	• Modified position changes little and often • Instability may be due to secretion retention, may respond well to gentle more frequent changes in position
Desaturation and long recovery post physiotherapy	• Perform physiotherapy carefully and separately from all cares
Signs of CO_2 retention, increased oxygen requirement with increased secretions	• Change position prophylactically; assess need for increased suction and chest techniques
Dislike by carers in the use of closed suction circuits	• Safer in oscillated babies and those on nitric oxide • Maintains pressures and PEEP • Prevents desaturations
Occasional inability to clear secretions with closed suction	• ETT may be small • Tube may be blocked • Change to open suction

CALL OUT TO NEONATAL PATIENT

What do you Need to Ask?
On the Telephone
• Has a chest X-ray been done?
• Blood gases, the trend? Stability of the infant and the mode of ventilation?
• Platelets, metabolic state (risk of congenital rickets)?

- Length of time since birth, respiratory history (respiratory distress syndrome/chronic lung disease, etc.)?

On the Ward
- Verbal handover.
- How the infant handles with carers/suctioning.
- Amounts of oxygen increase needed for this?
- Results of CXR?

From Charts/Monitors
- Gases, oxygenation HR, BP?
- Last series of care and effects?
- Nursed constantly in one position?
- Recent respiratory arrest/desaturations/bradycardias/ reintubations and the recorded cause?

Assessment
- Number of days from birth? If <7 then use positioning only.
- General response to handling?
- How frequently needing suctioning?
- Response generally to change of position?
- Colour, respiratory rate, etc.?
- Abdominal distension (modify position)?
- Cerebral bleeds?

Treatment Precautions

Remember:
If in doubt do NOT treat, discuss with team. If undertaking active techniques, the infant's head must always be fully supported, due to the risk of intra-cerebral bleeding.

- If the infant has neonatal rickets use positioning only.
- Avoid lying on clear lung for long periods of time with collapse on the other side, due to VQ mismatch.
- Always make note of acute medical state before embarking on active chest techniques, as the infant may be too unstable to cope with more than just a gentle change of position.

Treatment Contraindications
- Very sick unstable infant.
- Head down position – due to high incidence of reflux, this can cause increased cerebral pressure, increased intra-abdominal pressure in the presence of necrotizing enterocolitis.

- Very low platelets ($<50 \times 10^{-9}$) and/or if blood suctioned from ETT.
- Abdominal distension with necrotizing enterocolitis.
- Pulmonary haemorrhage.
- Pulmonary interstitial emphysema.
- Manual hyperinflation, risk of pneumothorax, barotraumas.

RISKS

Table 17.5 Consider the risks

Are you trained?	No:
	• If you feel confident, give simple advice on positioning and suction. If not suggest the paediatric anaesthetic team are called if the nursing staff are unable to treat the patient. Discuss the issue with the on call service manager the next working day
	Yes:
	• Refer to local guidelines for chest treatment in the preterm infant
	• NB: this includes local suctioning standards
	• Liaise with senior nursing/medical staff
Documentation	• Clear full, recording of assessment, treatment and advice given is essential
	• Leave a clear plan of recommendations for reassessment, changes of positioning and suctioning

TREATMENT TECHNIQUES

Table 17.6 Techniques and modifications

Treatment techniques	Modifications in neonates
Physiotherapy treatment	• Always treat with the nurse present to assist with alarms, suctioning, etc.
Positioning/postural drainage	• Head down contraindicated
	• Preferential ventilation of uppermost lung therefore VQ mismatch
	• Prone improves oxygenation, drains the posterior lung bases and is commonly the most stable position

	• Prone:
	  a. decreased reflux
	  b. decreased respiratory effort
	  c. better quality of sleep
	• Regular position changes within tolerance ensure no region of lung remains dependent for long periods of time

Manual hyperinflation	• **This is NOT used in the preterm infant** • Risk of pneumothorax • Does not utilize collateral ventilation as this is not established • Rescue/resuscitation only • Used in term or larger babies with caution
Percussion with Bennet face mask	• Head must be fully supported at all times • Always use appropriately sized mask • Follow local guidelines on appropriate pressures for percussion (0.5 cmH$_2$O in infants under 28 weeks) • Only treat in 1–2 positions at a time • Use 1–2 minutes of percussion in each position **stopping** if the infant desaturates or demonstrates poor tolerance • Suction when secretions have loosened • NB: small infants only tolerate two very short treatments with corresponding suctioning
Vibrations (done with the pad of the distal phalanx)	• Head must be fully supported at all times • Applied finely with 2–3 fingers throughout expiration, every 2–3 breaths • Used appropriately, 3–5 vibes will clear secretions and these can be felt mobilizing under the fingertips
Suctioning as an adjunct to physiotherapy	• In non-ventilated infants and those on nasal CPAP, clearance of the upper airway with nasopharyngeal suction is essential as infants are obligatory nose breathers

table continues

Treatment techniques	Modifications in neonates
Suctioning via ETT (should comply with local suctioning standard)	• Suction orally in ventilated babies; often secretions come around the tube • Complete suction in 8–10 seconds • Pressures 6–8 kPa • Catheter size only half the internal diameter of the ETT, e.g.: 2.5 = 5 3.0 = 6 • Only take the catheter 1 cm at the very most beyond the end of the ETT • Use saline in the following amounts: 23–28 weeks 0.2 ml 28–35 weeks 0.4 ml Term plus 0.5 ml

Remember:

It is imperative that wherever chest physiotherapy is practised, especially if this is shared by the nursing staff (i.e. respiratory care), the appropriate protocols, teaching and competency frameworks are in place to allow for accountability for any techniques being undertaken. This recorded information needs to be backed with full clinical reasoning and, wherever possible, evidence based practice protocols.

Key messages

- Only treat a neonatal patient if you are specifically trained in the care of neonates.
- If the baby is very small and fragile, with poor response to handling, maintain a hands-off approach.
- Try to avoid treatment in first week post birth (increased risk of cerebral bleed).
- If you are called to a neonatal patient and you are not trained in the physiotherapy management of neonates, do not treat the patient. It is better that the nursing staff continue to manage the patient. Contact a senior member of the medical, nursing or paediatric physiotherapy staff for support.

TREATMENT AND CASE STUDIES

CHAPTER 18 Respiratory physiotherapy treatments

Alison Draper and Paul Ritson

The following (alphabetical) list of treatment options will assist you in your treatment planning. Each individual patient will respond uniquely, therefore you may consider certain precautions or contra-indications appropriate in different circumstances. Safety and effective treatment must be your primary objectives.

Your scope of practice extends to treatment techniques that you have been trained to use. Do not undertake treatments for which you are not trained. It is your responsibility to request regular exposure to treatment techniques that you feel need practice.

ABDOMINAL BREATHING

See active cycle of breathing techniques (below).

ACTIVE CYCLE OF BREATHING TECHNIQUES (ACBT)

Cycle of deep breathing exercises (thoracic expansion exercises) and huffing (forced expiration technique – FET) interspersed with breathing control, used to aid clearance of secretions. Individual components can be used separately or emphasized within the cycle, depending on the patient's predominant symptoms (Fig. 18.1). May be used in conjunction with other treatments, e.g. manual techniques, positioning, etc.

ACBT – BREATHING CONTROL (BC) (Diaphragmatic breathing, abdominal breathing)

Tidal breathing, i.e. not deep breathing. The upper chest and shoulders should be relaxed.

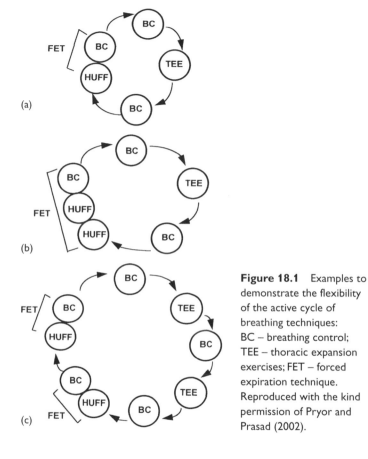

Figure 18.1 Examples to demonstrate the flexibility of the active cycle of breathing techniques: BC – breathing control; TEE – thoracic expansion exercises; FET – forced expiration technique. Reproduced with the kind permission of Pryor and Prasad (2002).

Table 18.1 Notes on ACBT – breathing control

	Adult	Child/baby
Indications	• Increased WOB • Shortness of breath • Altered breathing pattern • Panic attacks/anxiety • Hyperventilation	• Children as adult – may not cooperate • Babies n/a
Contraindications	• None	• None

Precautions	• Ensure patient is in a comfortable, well-supported position (see Positions of ease) • Check that the patient is not actively contracting their abdominals – movement of the abdomen should be passive	• As adult

Helpful Hints/Troubleshooting

- Encourage patients to breathe in through their nose (if appropriate) and to gently breathe out.
- A hand on the patient's abdomen can check for the desired rise and fall of the abdomen on inspiration and expiration. Be aware that for patients with less effective diaphragmatic activity this movement will be reduced.
- Use your calmest, most relaxing manner (see Relaxation).
- Ensure relaxation of the head, shoulder girdle and thorax.
- Give lots of encouragement, reassurance and praise.
- Do not expect fast results – patients who are experiencing shortness of breath are usually reluctant and/or unable (especially chronic chest patients) to change their breathing pattern quickly.
- Do not insist that the patient abandons bad breathing habits if the patient says they are helping.
- Do not tell patient to 'relax' or 'slow down their breathing' as this may increase anxiety.

ACBT – THORACIC EXPANSION EXERCISES (TEE)
(Deep breathing exercises, lateral costal breathing)

Maximal breath in followed by relaxed expiration. May be used in conjunction with manual techniques (e.g. percussion, vibrations or shaking) or inspiratory hold and/or sniff.

- Inspiratory hold: breath holding for a few seconds at the end of a deep breath in.
- Sniff: sniffing air in through the nose at the end of a deep breath in with the aim of recruiting collateral ventilation.

Table 18.2 Notes on ACBT – thoracic expansion exercises

	Adult	Child/baby
Indications	• Poor expansion due to collapse or atelectasis, pain, fear of pain or immobility • Sputum retention	• Children as adult • Babies n/a
Contraindications	• None	• None
Precautions	• Ensure that the patient has received adequate analgesia, if appropriate, before commencing treatment • Ensure that the patient is in a suitable position (see Positions to increase lung volume)	• As adult

Helpful Hints/Troubleshooting

- Use your hands to give firm support on the lateral aspects of the patient's ribcage (above the level of rib 8) to monitor the patient's performance and give some sensory input.
- Give lots of encouragement.
- Do not place your hands directly over an incision or painful area of the chest unless the patient is happy for you to do so.
- Do not ask the patient to perform more than three or four deep breaths at a time (may get dizzy).
- Patients who are breathless will not be able to perform consecutive TEEs. Intersperse TEEs with regular breathing control.

ACBT – FORCED EXPIRATION TECHNIQUE (FET) (Huff)

Gentle but forced breath out through an open mouth, following a breath in. The size of breath in will determine the level at which sputum clearance occurs.

Table 18.3 Notes on ACBT – forced expiration technique

	Adult	Child/baby
Indications	• Sputum retention	• Children as adult • Babies n/a
Contraindications	• None	• None
Precautions	• Bronchospasm	• As adult

Helpful Hints/Troubleshooting

- Spend time making sure the patient understands how to perform the technique effectively.
- Use analogies like 'steam up a mirror' to help your explanation.
- Encourage the patient to huff from a low lung volume, i.e. 'a small breath in' or 'half a breath in' initially, to mobilize peripheral secretions.
- Encourage the patient to huff from larger lung volumes, i.e. 'a deep breath in' to mobilize secretions in more proximal airways.
- The use of different lung volumes may help patients with overwhelming sputum production.
- Huff should be long enough to clear secretions, not simply a clearing of the throat, yet not so long as to lead into paroxysmal coughing.
- Intersperse forced expiration technique with breathing control.
- It can be difficult to teach children this technique. Try using peak flow mouthpiece or blowing games.

AUTOGENIC DRAINAGE

A cycle of breathing at different lung volumes which aims to produce high airflow in different lung regions in order to mobilize secretions. Needs to be taught to patients by physiotherapists who have had specific training in the technique.

Not a suitable technique to begin teaching in an on call situation, although some patients needing emergency physiotherapy may have been taught it previously. Do not attempt to instruct a patient in this technique unless you have been trained to do so.

Table 18.4 Notes on autogenic drainage

	Adult	Child/baby
Indications	• Sputum retention • Taught particularly to patients with chronic lung pathology	• Children as adult • Babies n/a
Contraindications	• None	• None
Precautions	• None	• None

Helpful Hints/Troubleshooting

- Only allow the patient to use this technique in the on call situation if they normally use it independently and they feel it is helpful.

BAGGING (Manual hyperinflation)

Deep breaths delivered manually to a mechanically ventilated patient by means of a rebreathing bag.

Table 18.5 Notes on bagging

	Adult	Child/baby
Indications	• Intubated patients with atelectasis or sputum retention	• As adults • Hypoxia
Contraindications	• Undrained pneumothorax • CVS instability/arrhythmias • Systolic BP <80 mmHg • Severe bronchospasm • Peak airway pressure >40 cmH$_2$O when mechanically ventilated • High PEEP requirement >15 cmH$_2$O • Unexplained haemoptysis	• Undrained pneumothorax • Severe bronchospasm • Severe CVS instability • Some cardiac conditions
Precautions	• Use a manometer to monitor peak pressures if available. Do not exceed 40 cmH$_2$O pressure • PEEP >10 cmH$_2$O – only bag if essential. Use PEEP valve while bagging if patient is PEEP dependent • Drained pneumothorax • Recent lung surgery (within last 14 days) • Arrhythmias or unstable BP • On 100% O$_2$ (FiO$_2$ = 1) – disconnection from the ventilator may cause sudden desaturation • Watch the monitor for changes in heart rate or blood pressure • Reduced respiratory drive – an air/oxygen mix may be preferable • Raised ICP	• High frequency oscillation – leave on ventilator as much as possible • Labile BP • Watch volume and pressure as pneumothorax easily happens

Slow deep inspiration will offer best physiological benefit (recruit collateral ventilation, improve re-expansion and ABGs).

An inspiratory hold at full inspiration will further recruit collateral ventilation (this is not helpful in patients prone to air trapping, e.g. emphysema).

A fast expiratory release will mimic FET and may stimulate a cough. It may be possible to maintain PEEP either held by hand or by means of a PEEP valve – do not try this on call unless you have been trained.

Helpful Hints/Troubleshooting:

- Use a 2 L bag for adults, a 500 ml open-ended bag for babies, 1 L bag for children.
- Paediatric bags have an open end valve – you will need to practice the technique of effectively and safely bagging this client group.
- Use a manometer when bagging paediatric patients – give approximately 10% above ventilator setting – positive inspiratory pressure/positive end expiratory pressure (PIP/PEEP).
- Do not bag a paediatric patient if you are inexperienced with this age group.
- If you are not confident bagging any patient ask the nurse to assist you by bagging while you undertake physiotherapy. This is a very appropriate use of resources.
- If possible, position the patient with the area of atelectasis or sputum retention uppermost. Side-lying is often the most appropriate position, but not always possible to achieve.
- Watch the patient's chest to assess expansion.
- Coordinate the procedure with the patient's own breathing if they are able to cooperate.
- Stop when audible secretions are heard.
- Do not give more than eight hyperinflations in succession; aim to mimic ACBT with no more than three or four.
- Do not continue if patient shows signs of distress, systolic blood pressure drops below 80 (in infants 55 mmHg, and 75 mmHg in children over 2 years), arrhythmias develop or ICP increases.

BREATHING CONTROL

See Active cycle of breathing.

CORNET (R.C.CORNET®)

Curved plastic tube with mouthpiece through which patient exhales producing positive expiratory pressure and vibration within the airways. Can be used in any position. Only consider using in on call setting if you are familiar with the technique and they are regularly used within your hospital.

Table 18.6 Notes on Cornet

	Adult	**Child/baby**
Indications	• Sputum retention	• Children as adult
		• Babies n/a
Contraindications	• None	• None
Precautions	• None	• None

Helpful Hints/Troubleshooting

• Patient should breathe out through Cornet at normal rate and depth.
• It is not possible to breathe in through a Cornet.
• Treatment time is estimated as 10–15 minutes or until chest is clear.

COUGH

Reflex or voluntary mechanism for clearing airways of secretions or foreign body. An effective breath in and closure of the glottis is required to generate enough expiratory velocity to create an effective cough.

Supported cough – cough with manual support from therapist's hands or pillow over incision or painful area such as fractured ribs.

Helpful Hints/Troubleshooting

• Ensure adequate pain relief has been given before commencing treatment.
• Allow the patient to sip a hot or cold drink intermittently during treatment if mouth is dry (unless NBM).

Table 18.7 Notes on cough

	Adult	**Child/baby**
Indications	• Prevention and treatment of sputum retention	• Children as adult • Babies n/a
Contraindications	• None	• As adult
Precautions	• Pain – ensure adequate analgesia • Severe bronchospasm – avoid paroxysmal coughing • Discourage unnecessary coughing in patients with significant frank haemoptysis, bleeding oesophageal varices, raised ICP either measured or suspected or recent cerebral bleed, major eye surgery	• Pertussis (whooping cough) – paroxysmal coughing can cause severe desaturation and bradycardia

- Ensure the patient is in a well supported position and leaning forward if possible, or with their knees drawn up towards their chest.
- Do not insist on repeated coughing if the patient is not productive.

COUGH – ASSISTED COUGH

Manual upwards compression of diaphragm given by therapist to replace the work of the abdominals in order to facilitate a cough in patients with spinal cord injury or neuromuscular disease (Fig. 18.2).

Helpful Hints/Troubleshooting

- If one person is assisting – place one hand on near side of chest the other on the opposite side with the forearm resting on the lower ribs (Fig. 18.2A).
- As the patient coughs the physiotherapist pushes in and up with the forearm and stabilizes the thorax with the hands.
- Or (Fig. 18.2B) both hands are placed on the lower thorax, with the elbows extended, and the physiotherapist pushes in and up with both arms.

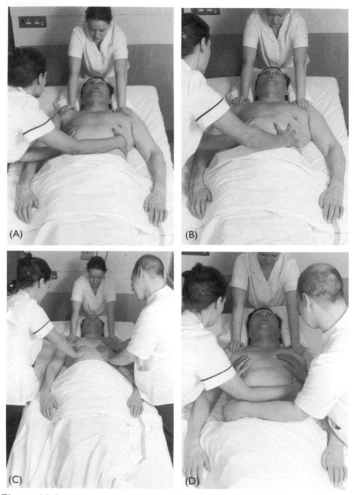

Figure 18.2 Assisted coughing. Reproduced with the kind permission of Pryor and Prasad (2002).

- In large patients or very tenacious sputum two people (Figs 18.2C and 18.2D) may be needed to effectively assist.
- Care is needed to synchronize the assisted cough with the patient's attempt to cough.

Table 18.8 Notes on assisted cough

	Adult	Child/baby
Indications	• Prevention and treatment of sputum retention	• Children as adult • Useful in children degenerative with neuromuscular disorders, e.g. Duchenne muscular dystrophy • Babies n/a
Contraindications	• Pressure on abdomen should be avoided as below, direct pressure over rib fractures of chest wall injuries/incisions should be avoided	• As adult
Precautions	• Immediately following surgery, especially post upper abdominal surgery, eye surgery, cardiothoracic surgery • Paralytic ileus • Rib fractures • Raised intracranial pressure • Undrained pneumothorax • Osteoporosis • Pain • Unstable spine – an appropriate hold must be used to counter any movement	• As adult

• Pressure should be released as soon as the cough is over.
• Patients with long-term cough assistance needs may have oped an effective interpretation of the above.

COUGH ASSIST DEVICE

Device which assists cough effort by means of a positive pre breath followed by a rapid switch to negative pressure. Most effe in patients who have an ineffective cough due to neuromuscular w ness. However, increasing use with other groups of patients.

Table 18.9 Notes on cough assist device

	Adult	Child/baby
Indications	• Prevention and treatment of sputum retention	• Children as adult • Babies n/a
Contraindications	• Undrained pneumothorax	• As adult
Precautions	• Oxygen dependency, entrain oxygen into the breathing circuit • Do not instigate use in the on call setting if you are not fully trained and confident • Bronchospasm	• As adult

Helpful Hints/Troubleshooting

- Fear, pain and poor technique will lead to poor synchrony with the machine and an ineffective treatment.
- A tight seal is essential – use either a face mask or a mouthpiece with nose clip; coughing is easier with a face mask if tolerated.
- Use as established with the patient – either the operator will synchronize the breath in and breath out to negative pressure with the patient, or the automatic mode may be used.
- Start with a low inspiratory pressure and gradually raise the pressure to achieve a deep breath with the patient (if on NIV start at the level set on the ventilator), initially keep inspiratory and expiratory pressure equal. Then increase expiratory pressure if the patient needs more 'suck'. Refer to your unit policy.

The patient is instructed to cough when the breath out starts.

- The technique can be combined with an assisted cough.
- The patient may need a few inspiratory breaths post coughing to recover.

COUGH STIMULATION/TRACHEAL RUB

This is a highly contentious issue – only use the technique if you are trained in its use and it is accepted practice within your hospital. Children over 18 months may mimic coughing, unwell children are less inclined to cooperate. Expectoration is rare before 3–4 years. Tracheal compression can stimulate a cough. Gentle pressure is applied to the trachea below the thyroid cartilage, stimulating a cough reflex. Care is needed with small infants due to the risk of bradycardia.

CONTINUOUS POSITIVE AIRWAY PRESSURE (CPAP)

Continuous positive pressure delivered throughout inspiration and expiration administered to a spontaneously breathing patient. Requires a high oxygen flow rate, delivered via an airtight mask, mouthpiece (with nose clip), trache or ET tube (Fig. 18.3). Can be given periodically or continuously.

Helpful Hints/Troubleshooting

- Oxygen and pressure levels should be set in liaison with medical staff. Do not try to set up this equipment unless you have been shown how to do so. Ask for assistance from ICU.
- Patients on CPAP generally require higher dependency care – check hospital policy with the ward sister.
- Other types of treatment such as breathing exercises can still be used with patients who are breathing with the assistance of CPAP.

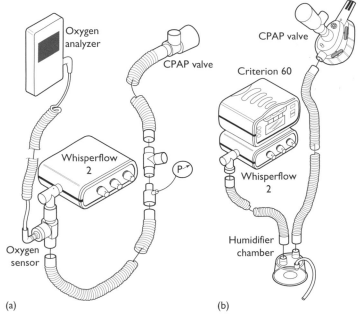

(a) (b)

Figure 18.3 Diagram to show an example of a CPAP circuit. Reproduced with the kind permission of Profile Systems Ltd.

Table 18.10 Notes on CPAP

	Adult	Child/baby
Indications	• Increased WOB or hypoxaemia caused by atelectasis, reduced FRC, flail chest, poor gas exchange across the basement membrane due to inflammation, pulmonary oedema, chronic damage	• As adults
Contraindications	• Undrained pneumothorax • Frank haemoptysis • Vomiting • Facial fractures, nasal approach for neurosurgery • CVS instability • Raised ICP • Recent upper GI surgery • Active TB • Lung abscess	• As adults
Precautions	• Increasing $PaCO_2$ • Emphysema – check CXR for large bullae • Patient compliance • Skin around mask can break down easily • Patients with airways obstructed by a tumour – may cause air trapping • Deranged platelets	• As adults. Children tend to dislike the sealed mask • Watch the amount of CPAP given – too much can cause increased WOB • Start at $4\,cmH_2O$ and assess patient closely

Monitor the patient's oxygen saturation if you need to remove the patient's mask for any reason, e.g. in order for them to cough.
- The beneficial effects of the CPAP are lost within minutes of removal – thus it may be in the patient's best interests to stay on CPAP. However, it may be appropriate, once stabilized, to enable the patient to have short periods of time without the CPAP for personal hygiene, skin care and a drink.
- Humidification is recommended.

- Be aware that CPAP will not correct a climbing $PaCO_2$ in adults but can sometimes be effective in infants under 1 year old.

DEEP BREATHING EXERCISES

See Active cycle of breathing techniques.

DIAPHRAGMATIC BREATHING

See Active cycle of breathing techniques.

FLUTTER

Pipe-shaped device through which the patient exhales past a ball-bearing, producing pressure oscillations in the airways. Can be used alone or in conjunction with other techniques.

Table 18.11   Notes on flutter

	Adult	Child/baby
Indications	• Sputum retention	• Children as adult
		• Babies n/a
Contraindications	• None	• None
Precautions	• None	• None

Helpful Hints/Troubleshooting

- Not first line emergency treatment, but do allow patients to use the flutter if they have already been given one and feel it is helpful.
- Make sure that maximal oscillation is achieved by adjusting the angle at which the flutter is held.
- Most easily used in sitting.
- Ensure that the patient is still doing TEEs and mobilizing as appropriate.

FORCED EXPIRATION TECHNIQUE (FET)

See Active cycle of breathing techniques.

GRAVITY ASSISTED POSITIONING/DRAINAGE

See Positioning.

HUFF

See Active cycle of breathing techniques – FET.

HUMIDIFICATION

Inhaled water vapour or aerosol administered by mask.

Table 18.12 Notes on humidification

	Adult	Child/baby
Indications	• Sputum retention, particularly thick sticky secretions, difficulty expectorating, dry mouth • Patients needing continuous oxygen (oxygen is a dry gas) • Patients breathing via a tracheostomy/ET tube (the natural warming mechanism of the nasal passages is bypassed)	• As adult
Contraindications	• None	• None
Precautions	• Patients prone to bronchospasm may react to nebulized water. Use saline if required – this will reduce the lifespan of the humidification unit as the saline will crystallize • Airway/facial burns if heated humidification is unmonitored (all new equipment should have temperature gauges and alarms)	• Can exacerbate fluid overload in cardiac conditions • Given via head box in infants and mask in children

Helpful Hints/Troubleshooting

• Many different types of equipment available. Make sure you are familiar with the type your unit uses.

- Using the bubble through method to humidify via nasal cannulae will return gas to atmospheric humidification but will not increase it, the water tends to condense in the narrow tubing. Wide diameter tubing and mask are essential for effective delivery.
- Give humidification time to have an effect. Ideally, if indicated, ask for it to be commenced before you arrive on the scene. If you commence humidification as part of your treatment allow approximately 10–15 minutes before recommencing sputum clearance techniques.
- Cold air blowing onto heated humidification tubing (e.g. fans, open windows) will cause water to collect in the tubing – this should be emptied regularly and ideally avoided.
- Due to the potential for infection, humidification units should not be left switched off and then reused.
- Also consider regular saline nebulizers and appropriate systemic hydration.

INCENTIVE SPIROMETER

Device which gives visual feedback on performance of slow deep breath in.

Table 18.13   Notes on incentive spirometer

	Adult	Child/baby
Indications	• Volume loss. May be useful for patients who have difficulty with understanding the concept of TEEs	• Children as adult. Limited to use by older children • Babies n/a
Contraindications	• None	• None
Precautions	• None	• None

Helpful Hints/Troubleshooting

- Give clear instructions. Patients need to be able to remember how to use the device so that they can use it when you are not there.
- Encourage the patient to adopt a position which will facilitate deep breathing (see Positioning to increase lung volume).
- Be aware that patients can quickly learn to cheat – ensure that what you are seeing is indeed the product of a slow deep breath in.
- Unhelpful for patients who are breathless.
- Cannot be used with patients who require a high concentration of continuous oxygen by mask.

INTERMITTENT POSITIVE PRESSURE BREATHING (IPPB)
(e.g. 'Bird', Bennet PR2)

Device which delivers positive pressure on inspiration only, to increase tidal volume and rest respiratory muscles, delivery is by mouthpiece or face mask (Fig. 18.4).

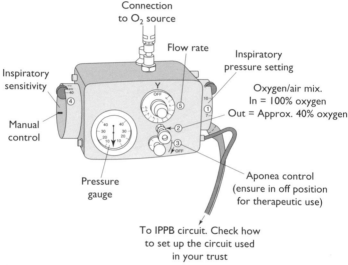

Figure 18.4 Diagram to show an example of IPPB dials.

Helpful Hints/Troubleshooting
- Position the patient with the area of volume loss or retained secretions area uppermost if possible.
- Adult settings for IPPB where numbered dials are present:
  a. sensitivity – keep low at approx 7, unless the machine appears to be triggering too easily.
  b. flow rate – start at 10 unless patient is very breathless. If very SOB start higher (over 20) and be prepared to quickly adjust it until the breath in is fast enough for the patient.
  c. pressure – start at 10 and aim to increase as able within the limits of the patient during the treatment.
- In paediatric patients, DO NOT use if the patient is uncompliant or under 5 years old.

Table 18.14 Notes on IPPB

	Adult	Child/baby
Indications	• Increased WOB, sputum retention, poor tidal volume particularly in weak or tired patients	• As adult. • Children older than 6 years of age seem to be able to comply
Contraindications	• Undrained pneumothorax • Frank haemoptysis • Vomiting blood (haematemesis) • Facial fractures, nasal approach for neurosurgery • CVS instability • Raised ICP • Recent lung/upper GI surgery • Active TB • Lung abscess	• As adult
Precautions	• Emphysema – check CXR for bullae • Patients with airways obstructed by a tumour – may cause air trapping • Deranged platelets	• As adult

- Suggested starting pressures for paediatric patients are as follows :
  a. $10\,cmH_2O$ then increase to $20\text{–}25\,cmH_2O$ maximum
- Pay attention to ensuring that after triggering the machine the rest of the inspiratory phase is passive – the patient must allow the machine to do the work of inspiration.
- Ensure that the patient is reaching the set pressure. If the pressure dial swings above the set pressure level, it is likely that the patient is blowing out into the machine – the machine will cut out early and the set pressure will not actually be achieved.
- Use saline in the machine's nebulizer.
- An effective seal is essential, either by means of a tight seal with the face mask (you will need to make sure that the head is supported so that you can hold the mask securely in place), or use a mouthpiece and pinch the nose. A nose clip may be useful for some patients.
- Use for short periods of time, not continuously, e.g. 10 minutes every hour. Remember not to give the patient more than about four

to eight big breaths in a row. If the nursing staff are to assist the patient it is essential that they are familiar with the equipment, the risk of pneumothorax, and are aware not to change the settings.

- Do not allow the patient to use the machine unsupervised unless you are confident they can use it effectively.
- Regularly seek exposure to IPPB as part of your learning to stay familiar with the machine and the appropriate settings to use.
- If everything is going wrong and you lose confidence with the bird as you start your treatment, take the machine away and, with a clean circuit, use the machine on yourself to sort out the cause of any problem, then return to the patient and start again.
- If IPPB is not available to you treat the patient with the physiotherapy techniques you consider most appropriate and inform the medical staff if further assistance beyond physiotherapy is needed.

LATERAL COSTAL BREATHING

See Active cycle of breathing techniques.

MANUAL HYPERINFLATION

See Bagging.

MOBILIZATION

Assisted walking or other functional activity such as moving from bed to chair. Most patients requiring on call physiotherapy will not be well enough to mobilize.

Table 18.15 Notes on mobilization

	Adult	Child/baby
Indications	• Sputum retention • Volume loss • Limited to previously mobile patients	• Children as adult • A toddler may need assistance to mobilize • Babies – ensure that the baby is able to roll and move around the cot – THIS IS STILL MOBILIZING THE PATIENT!

| Contraindications | • CVS instability
• Low BP, serious arrhythmia | • As adult |
| Precautions | • Drips, drains and catheters
• Ensure pain controlled
• Follow local protocols for patients with epidural analgesia, post orthopaedic, plastic, vascular surgery, etc. | • As adult |

Helpful Hints/Troubleshooting

• Ensure you get sufficient help before attempting to help a patient get out of bed.

• Work with the patient enabling them to assist in the manoeuvre as much as possible.

• The child in pain will be reluctant to mobilize. Ensure adequate analgesia and utilize all your powers of persuasion and bribery!

NEUROPHYSIOLOGICAL FACILITATION OF RESPIRATION

The selective use of external proprioceptive and tactile stimuli to produce a reflex respiratory response, with the aim of improving an aspect of ventilatory activity. These techniques are appropriate for on call treatments only if you are familiar with their effective use.

NON-INVASIVE VENTILATION (NIV)

Device which provides ventilatory support by delivering a pre-set volume or pressure by mask either automatically or in response to patient's inspiratory effort. Some machines are able to add positive end expiratory pressure.

Table 18.16   Notes on NIV

	Adult	**Child/baby**
Indications	• Increased WOB causing ventilatory failure, i.e. increased CO_2, fatigue, neuromuscular disorders	• As adult • Not often used in infants – nasal CPAP more commonly used

table continues

	Adult	Child/baby
Contraindications	• Undrained pneumothorax • Frank haemoptysis • Vomiting blood (haematemesis) • Facial fractures • CVS instability • Raised ICP • Recent upper GI surgery • Active TB • Lung abscess	• As adults

Precautions	• Emphysema – check
	  CXR for bullae
	• Patient compliance
	• Skin around mask can break
	  down easily
	• Patients with airways
	  obstructed by a tumour –
	  may cause air trapping
		• As adults
		• Children may dislike
		  the tight sealed mask

Helpful Hints/Troubleshooting

- Do not set up NIV unless you are familiar with the equipment, circuits, masks, etc. and are confident as to how safely to establish the patient on NIV and appropriately respond to blood gas results.
- The decision to use NIV and the settings chosen must always be made with the medical and nursing team looking after the patient.
- Introduce the treatment to the patient slowly.
- Patient needs to keep mouth closed if using nasal mask.
- Some patients are less suited to NIV; however, each situation should be individually assessed.
- NIV should generally be used in ICU/HDU environments – make sure you are aware of your local policy.

The steps in initiating NIV therapy. Reproduced with the kind permission of Pryor and Prasad (2002).

- Introduce the patient slowly to the equipment and all its parts.
- Ensure the mask fits comfortably and that the patient can experience the mask on their face without the ventilator connected.
- Allow the patient the opportunity to feel the operation of the machine through the mask on their hand or cheek before applying it over their nose or mouth.

- Allow the patient the opportunity to practise breathing with the ventilator, either holding the mask in place or allowing them to hold it in place before applying the straps.
- Adjust settings initially for comfort and establish whether the patient can relax comfortably in a sleeping posture.
- Provide opportunities for the patient to feed back any discomfort or uncertainty with regard to the use of the equipment.
- Assess and adjust the performance of the ventilator during an afternoon nap to optimize gas exchange and patient comfort.
- Progress to an overnight study, continuing to monitor and optimize gas exchange and sleep quality.

Characteristics of patients with acute respiratory failure unlikely to do well on NIV:
Reproduced with the kind permission of Pryor and Prasad (2002).

- Agitation, encephalopathic, uncooperative
- Severe illness, including extreme acidosis (pH <7.2)
- Presence of excessive secretions or pneumonia
- Multiple organ failure
- Haemodynamic instability
- Inability to maintain a lip seal
- Inability to protect the airway
- Overt respiratory failure requiring immediate intubation

OVERPRESSURE

Applied at the end of the breath out and is quickly released to stimulate inspiration. Only appropriate in the paralysed patient. Care is needed in patients with chest trauma/post surgery and fragile ribs, e.g. osteoporosis.

OXYGEN THERAPY

Delivery of higher concentration of oxygen than is present in room air, i.e. 24–100% by mask, nasal canulae, ET tube, etc.

Should be prescribed in writing by a doctor in adults but given as necessary without prescription in paediatrics unless there is an underlying duct-dependent cardiac lesion. Any change (beyond appropriate pre-oxygenation for suction) must be discussed with the medical team.

Toxic if given in high concentrations over prolonged period.

Table 18.17 Notes on oxygen therapy

	Adult	Child/baby
Indications	• Hypoxaemia • Before and after suction	• As adult
Contraindications	• None	• Duct-dependent cardiac lesions – follow local protocols
Precautions	• Hypercapnic COPD patients who may be dependent on hypoxaemia for respiratory drive. Use ABGs to assess – see Chapter 4	• Remember humidification if over 2 L/minute given

Helpful Hints/Troubleshooting

- Ensure adequate humidification is provided with continuous use of high concentrations.
- Avoid prolonged patient exposure to unnecessarily high concentrations.

PEP MASK (POSITIVE EXPIRATORY PRESSURE MASK)

Mask which provides resistance to expiration, to facilitate sputum clearance and improve lung volume.

Table 18.18 Notes on PEP mask

	Adult	Child/baby
Indications	• Sputum retention	• Children as adult • Babies n/a
Contraindications	• None	• None
Precautions	• None	• Younger children may dislike sealed mask

Helpful Hints/Troubleshooting

- Do not initiate use unless you are familiar with the device.
- Allow patients to use the PEP mask if they have been given one and feel it is helpful.
- Allow the patient to hold the mask themselves and make sure they maintain an airtight seal against the face.

- If a manometer is used the pressure should be between 10 and 20 cmH$_2$O during mid-expiration.
- Generally used in forward lean sitting with elbows on the table, holding the mask firmly over the mouth and nose (a mouthpiece and nose clip may be used).
- Tidal volume breathing with a slightly active expiration for 6–10 breaths.
- Treatment length is approximately 15 minutes and FET is used intermittently.
- In an acute exacerbation some chronic sputum producers, e.g. cystic fibrosis or bronchiectasis, may need some extra help with sputum clearance – this is best discussed with the patient/carers/medical team.

PERCUSSION

Rhythmic clapping on the patient's chest with cupped hands or soft-rimmed face mask.

Table 18.19   Notes on percussion

	Adult	Child/baby
Indications	• Sputum retention	• As adult
Contraindications	• Directly over rib fracture • Directly over a surgical incision or graft • Frank haemoptysis • Severe osteoporosis	• Hypoxia – percussion can exacerbate hypoxia, especially in infants
Precautions	• Profound hypoxaemia • Bronchospasm, pain • Osteoporosis, bony metastases • Near chest drains	• As adult • **Baby – make sure head is supported**

Helpful Hints/Troubleshooting

- For adults and older children perform in conjunction with thoracic expansion exercises.
- To minimize hypoxaemia percussion during TEEs (i.e. approximately 30 seconds) is recommended.
- Cushion the patient with a folded towel, and be careful not to be heavy handed – patient comfort is important.

POSITIONING – POSITIONS OF EASE

Well supported patient positions used with spontaneously breathing patients which encourage relaxation of the upper chest and shoulders (Fig. 18.5).

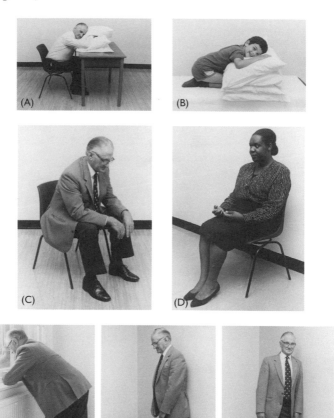

Figure 18.5 Positions of ease. **A.** Forward lean sitting. **B.** Forward kneeling. **C and D.** Relaxed sitting. **E.** Forward lean standing. **F and G.** Relaxed standing. Reproduced with the kind permission of Pryor and Prasad (2002).

Table 18.20 Notes on positions of ease

	Adult	**Child/baby**
Indications	• Increased WOB • SOB at rest and on exercise • Anxiety/panic attacks • Hyperventilation	• Children as adult • Babies (see Fig. 18.5B)
Contraindications	• None	• None
Precautions	• None	• None

POSITIONING – POSTURAL DRAINAGE (Gravity assisted drainage)

Positions which allow gravity to help drain retained secretions (see Fig. 18.6 and Table 18.21 for exact positions).

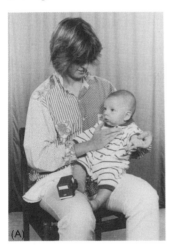

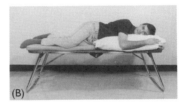

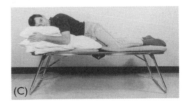

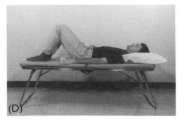

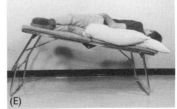

Figure 18.6 (caption overleaf).

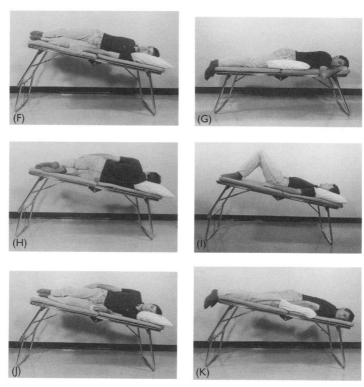

Figure 18.6 Postural drainage. **A.** Apical segments upper lobes. **B.** Posterior segment right upper lobe. **C.** Posterior segment left upper lobe. **D.** Anterior segments upper lobes. **E.** Lingula. **F.** Right middle lobe. **G.** Apical segments lower lobes. **H.** Right medial basal and left lateral basal segments lower lobes. **I.** Anterior basal segments. **J.** Lateral basal segment right lower lobe. **K.** Posterior basal segments lower lobes. Reproduced with the kind permission of Pryor and Prasad (2002).

Table 18.21 Notes on postural drainage

	Adult	**Child/baby**
Indications	• Sputum retention, particularly if localized to one lung segment or lobe	• As adult

Contraindications to head down position	• Hypertension • Severe dyspnoea • Recent surgery • Severe haemoptysis • Nose bleeds • Advanced pregnancy • Hiatus hernia • Cardiac failure • Cerebral oedema • Aortic aneurysm • Head or neck trauma/ surgery • Mechanical ventilation	• As adult
Precautions	• Diaphragmatic paralysis/ weakness	• Head down position can cause reflux, vomiting and aspiration

Table 18.22 Gravity assisted drainage positions (Prasad and Pryor 2002)

	Lobe	Position
Upper lobe	• Apical bronchus • Posterior bronchus • Right	• Sitting upright • Lying on the left side horizontally turned 45° on to the face, resting against a pillow, with another supporting the head
	• Left	• Lying on the right side turned 45° on to the face, with three pillows arranged to lift the shoulders 30 cm from the horizontal
	• Anterior bronchus	• Lying supine with the knees flexed
Lingula	• Superior brochus • Inferior bronchus	• Lying supine with the body a quarter turned to the right maintained by a pillow under the left side from shoulder to hip. The chest is tilted downwards to an angle of 15°
Middle lobe	• Lateral bronchus • Medial bronchus	• Lying supine with the body a quarter turned to the left

table continues

Lobe	Position
	maintained by a pillow under the right side from shoulder to hip. The chest is tilted downwards to an angle of 15°
Lower lobe • Apical bronchus	• Lying prone with a pillow under the abdomen
• Medial basal (cardiac) bronchus	• Lying on the right side with the chest tilted downwards to an angle of 20°
• Anterior basal bronchus	• Lying supine with the knees flexed and the chest tilted downwards to an angle of 20°
• Lateral basal bronchus	• Lying on the opposite side with the chest tilted downwards to an angle of 20°
• Posterior basal bronchus	• Lying prone with a pillow under the hips and the chest tilted downwards to an angle of 20°

Helpful Hints/Troubleshooting

- Do not use head down tilt immediately after meals/feed.
- Position needs to be maintained for at least 10 minutes to achieve a beneficial effect.
- Can be modified to side-lying (affected lung uppermost) with or without head down tip for more generalized secretions or those with contraindications to head down position.
- Drain worst affected area first.
- Most hospital beds have a catch at the bottom of the bed or an electric switch which will tip the bed feet up.
- Especially in children positioning for drainage may result in a VQ mismatch. Discuss this with the medical team. It may be necessary to either adapt the position or temporarily increase the oxygen.

POSITIONING TO INCREASE VOLUME

Positioning spontaneously breathing patients to facilitate maximal inspiration. Usually involves use of upright positions – standing, high sitting or side lying.

Table 18.23 Notes on positioning to increase volume

	Adult	Child/baby
Indications	• Volume loss, i.e. poor expansion due to pain, fear of pain, immobility	• As adult
Contraindications	• CVS instability • Unstable spinal fracture • Unstable head injury	• As adult
Precautions	• Proceed slowly if standing the patient for the first time after a period of bed rest	• As adult

Helpful Hints/Troubleshooting

• Get as much help as you need to move the patient safely.

POSITIONING TO MATCH VENTILATION/ PERFUSION RATIO

Positioning which attempts to maximally perfuse and ventilate the same area of healthy lung tissue. Best applied to patients with unilateral pathology.

Table 18.24 Notes on positioning to match ventilation/perfusion ratio

	Adult	Child/baby
Indications	• Hypoxaemia	• As adult
Contraindications	• As above (Table 18.23)	• As adult
Precautions	• As above	• As adult
Ventilated	• Lung with pathology down	• Lung with pathology up (baby and small child)
Non-ventilated	• Lung with pathology up	• Lung with pathology down (baby and small child)

Helpful Hints/Troubleshooting

• Get as much help as you need to move the patient safely.
• Ensure that you are happy with principles of ventilation and perfusion before deciding how to position the patient – dependent regions of lung are preferentially ventilated and perfused in spontaneously breathing adults.
• Babies, small children and mechanically ventilated adults ventilate non-dependent lung regions while perfusing dependent regions and it is therefore difficult to match ventilation and perfusion.

POSITIONING – PRONE

Profoundly hypoxic patients may be nursed prone as this aids the recruitment of lung tissue. Chest physiotherapy is still possible in this position if appropriate. Most patients requiring this intervention do not have sputum retention as a problem and require high levels of PEEP and oxygen and may thus not benefit from physiotherapy.

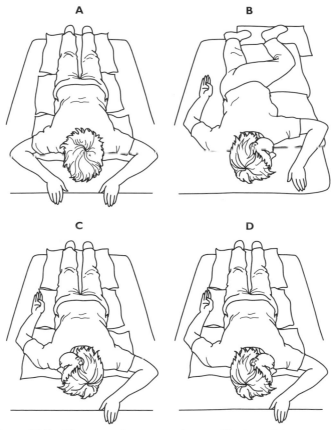

A   B

C   D

Figure 18.7   Diagram to show appropriate modifications of the prone position to individualize to the patient's shape, pressure area care and protection of the neuro-musculoskeletal structures. Adapted with kind permission of Ball et al (2001).

However, be aware of the need to protect neural and soft tissues. See Figure 18.7 for suggested upper limb positioning.

This position is used commonly in paediatrics due to its beneficial effect on gas exchange. If you utilize this position, make sure that the patient is **carefully monitored** (i.e. HR, BP, SpO_2, RR) owing to the link with sudden infant death syndrome.

POSITIVE EXPIRATORY PRESSURE MASK

See PEP mask.

POSTURAL DRAINAGE

See Positioning.

RELAXATION TECHNIQUES

Techniques which help patients reduce unhelpful muscle tension. May include appropriate use of voice, calm manner, advice on positioning, advice on breathing and specific relaxation techniques such as 'Laura Mitchell', or 'contract/relax'.

Table 18.25   Notes on relaxation techniques

	Adult	Child/baby
Indications	• Increased WOB • SOB at rest and on exercise • Altered breathing pattern • Panic attacks, anxiety • Hyperventilation	• Children as adult • Babies n/a
Contraindications	• None	• None
Precautions	• None	• None

Helpful Hints/Troubleshooting

• Never underestimate the power of relaxation: simple positioning, use of voice and reassurance can have a profound impact upon anxiety related increase WOB and bronchospasm.

• Ensure that you are relaxed yourself if you intend to try to reduce tension in your patient.

• Position the patient appropriately – forward lean sitting or high side-lying are useful.

- Incorporate appropriate aspects of relaxation into managing the breathing problem.
- Be aware that a noisy bustling ward will reduce the efficacy of your treatment!

RELAXED TIDAL BREATHING

See Active cycle of breathing techniques.

RIB SPRINGING

Used in the paralysed patient. Compression of the chest wall is continued throughout expiration with the application of overpressure at the end of expiration. A quick release stimulates inspiration.

Care is required at the level of compression offered as the patient is unable to report pain. Do not use unless familiar with the technique. Contraindicated for babies and all patients with fragile ribs/vertebrae (e.g. osteoporosis).

SHAKING

Coarse oscillations produced by the therapist's hands compressing and releasing the chest wall. Performed during thoracic expansion exercises, on exhalation only.

Table 18.26 Notes on shaking

	Adult	Child/baby
Indications Contraindications	• Sputum retention • Directly over rib fracture or surgical incision	• Sputum retention • Premature infants – causes brain injury – DO NOT USE
Precautions	• Long-term oral steroids/ osteoporosis, bony metastases • Near chest drains • Severe bronchospasm	• Rib fractures • **Baby – make sure head is supported**

Helpful Hints/Troubleshooting

- Perform on the expiration phase only following a deep breath in.
- Obtain feedback from the patient concerning comfort – this technique should not be uncomfortable.

SPUTUM INDUCTION (Induced sputum)

Use of nebulized (via ultrasonic nebulizer) hypertonic saline concentrations to facilitate expectoration of sputum specimen. Bronchospasm is a risk – access to prescribed bronchodilators is essential.

Not generally an indication for emergency physiotherapy – you will not be able to access the equipment or be skilled in its use. Check if the call out is still appropriate for physiotherapy treatment.

SUCTION – ENDOTRACHEAL SUCTION

Removal of secretions from the upper airways using a suction catheter, in patients who are intubated or have a tracheostomy.

Table 18.27 Notes on endotracheal suction

	Adult	Child/baby
Indications	• Sputum retention in intubated patients • Sputum retention may be indicated by high peak airway pressures with volume controlled ventilation or decreased tidal volume with pressure controlled ventilation, auscultation, hypoxaemia or reduced SpO_2	• Sputum retention indicated by raised heart rate in association with other indications • Decreased SpO_2/hypoxia • Deteriorating blood gases in association with other indications • Increased WOB • Auscultation in association with other indications • Visible/audible secretions not effectively removed with a cough and causing respiratory distress • Poor cough caused by neurological pathology, pain inhibition, or inhibition by drugs • Aspiration • Reduced tidal volumes in ventilated patients

table continues

	Adult	Child/baby
Contraindications Precautions	• None if indicated • Low SpO_2 • Dependency on high O_2 • High ventilatory requirements (closed circuit catheters will reduce need to disconnect patient from ventilator) • Severe CVS instability • Anticoagulated patients or those with clotting disorders • Severe bronchospasm • Recent lung oesophageal surgery	• Increased peak pressures in vented patients • As adult • As adult

Helpful Hints/Troubleshooting

- Preoxygenate before and after suction either by bagging or by increasing the baseline FiO_2 on the ventilator by:
  a. 10% for children/babies
  b. 20% or up to 100% depending upon unit policy for adults.
- Use each catheter only once unless closed system suction is used.
- Discontinue if arrhythmias develop, or HR/BP drop.
- Explain the procedure to the patient with lots of reassurance.
- Suction catheter size – internal diameter of tube × 2, minus 2 = size of suction catheter, e.g. tube size 7 = (7 × 2) − 2 = 12.

SUCTION – PHARYNGEAL SUCTION

Removal of secretions from the upper airways by means of a suction catheter introduced via the nose or mouth. Generally only indicated for patients who are unconscious/semiconscious or neurologically impaired. (See section on consent, Ch. 1, p. 7.)

Table 18.28   Notes on pharyngeal suction

	Adult	Child/baby
Indications	• Retained secretions/ aspiration in the upper airways of patients who are unable to cough or have reduced cough caused by fatigue, neurological pathology, pain inhibition, or inhibition by drugs	• Visible/audible secretions not effectively removed with a cough and causing respiratory distress • Poor cough caused by neurological pathology, pain inhibition, or inhibition by drugs • Aspiration
Contraindications	• Stridor • Skull fractures • Craniofacial surgery/injury	• Haemangioma • As adult
Precautions	• High malignancy, high oesophageal varices • Anticoagulated patients or those with clotting disorders • Severe CVS instability • Severe bronchospasm • Recent pneumonectomy or oesophagectomy – liaise with surgeons	• As adult

Helpful Hints/Troubleshooting

- Use an airway for oral suction or frequent nasal suctioning.
- Preoxygenate the patient.
- Position the patient in side-lying in case they vomit.
- Use a 'clean' technique.
- Do not use on any patient who would require physical restraining in order to carry out the procedure.
- Do not suction patients to remove pulmonary oedema as it will be replaced and surfactant will be removed.
- Remember to give the patient lots of reassurance.
- Some units will insert a mini tracheostomy (a thin blue tube) into the trachea if repeated suction is needed. This procedure is associated

with as much risk as formal tracheostomy insertion and thus the decision is not taken lightly (see Ch. 12).
- Mini tracheostomy is not used in the majority of paediatric units.

THORACIC EXPANSION EXERCISES

See Active cycle of breathing techniques.

VIBRATIONS

Fine oscillations applied to the chest wall by the therapist's hands or fingertips (in babies). Performed during thoracic expansion exercises, on exhalation only.

Table 18.29 Notes on vibrations

	Adult	Child/baby
Indications	• Sputum retention	• Sputum retention
Contraindications	• Directly over rib fracture or surgical incision • Severe bronchospasm	• Premature infants – causes brain injury if head is unsupported
Precautions	• Long-term oral steroids/ osteoporosis • Near chest drains	• Rib fractures • Make sure head is supported

Helpful Hints/Troubleshooting
- Use firm contact and direct the force inwards towards the centre of the patient's chest.
- Perform on the expiration phase only following a deep breath in.

References

Ball C, Adams J, Boyce S et al (2001) Clinical guidelines for the use of the prone position in acute respiratory distress syndrome. Intensive Crit Care Nurs 17(2):94–104.

Pryor JA, Prasad SA (eds) (2002) Physiotherapy for respiratory and cardiac problems, 3rd edn. London: Churchill Livingstone.

Further reading

Hough A (2001) Physiotherapy in respiratory care, 3rd edn. Cheltenham: Stanley Thornes.

CHAPTER 19 **Case studies**

This chapter contains a number of case studies written by the authors of the chapters in Section 3. Work through the ones specific to your learning needs. Do not worry if the information given or presentation differs – this is all part of the learning process.

CASE STUDY 1 – ADULT INTENSIVE CARE UNIT

Rachel Devlin

A 65-year-old man was admitted with 3-day history of increased shortness of breath, persistent pyrexia and green sputum. He deteriorated in A&E requiring intubation and ventilation and was transferred to the intensive care unit.

History

PMH: Mild asthma
DH: Ventolin inhaler p.r.n.
SH: Lives with wife; smokes 20 cigarettes a day

You are called to see this patient due to deterioration in PaO_2 and difficulty in obtaining secretions.

On Examination

Patient is intubated via an oral ETT, and has recently been positioned in left side-lying.

Ventilation
PS 20   PEEP 12   Respiratory rate 32
TV =350 ml (previously 550 ml)   MV = 11.2 L
PAP 25 cmH$_2$O FiO$_2$ 0.5 SpO$_2$ 92% (previously 98%)
ABGs   pH 7.35 PaCO$_2$ 4.5
              PaO$_2$ 8.3 HCO$_3^-$ 22
              BE −1
CVS   HR 110 BP 100/60

Urine output = 40 ml per hour
Temperature 38.5°C
Drugs: Propofol, fentanyl, noradrenaline (norepinephrine)
Auscultation: Absent breath sounds left lower lobe
Minimal purulent secretions during last hour

Questions:
1 What is the patient's main problem? What additional information may you require?
2 What is your treatment plan?
3 What precautions/contraindications do you need to consider prior to treatment?

Answer 1:
- Desaturation following turning into left side-lying, as a result of a sputum plug.
- Preferential ventilation occurs in the uppermost lung and perfusion is optimal in the dependent lung. In this case, the left lower lobe is collapsed and is receiving preferential perfusion but is not ventilated, causing a decrease in SpO_2.
- It is also important to consider that despite cardiac support drugs the patient's BP is low; this may have an impact upon your physiotherapy treatment.
- A new CXR would assist your assessment.

Answer 2:
- Position the patient in right side-lying to optimize ventilation to the left lung.
- Along with suction, consider saline instilled via the ETT, saline nebulizer, manual techniques and heated humidification to increase sputum clearance.
- Also consider using a closed suction system to minimize the side-effects of suction, e.g. loss of PEEP.

Answer 3:
- Positioning may lower blood pressure; therefore it is vital that the physiotherapist observes the bedside monitors (ECG and BP) at all times. Introduce each treatment technique individually and carefully and then reassess. If blood pressure initially drops this may be

transient and rectify itself; however, if it persists the patient may require further medical management and perhaps repositioning in supine to improve BP. Physiotherapy treatment may therefore have to take place in a less than optimal position, or once the patient has settled.

- Manual hyperinflation is cautioned against for patients with PEEP >10 cmH$_2$O.
- Manual hyperinflation may cause blood pressure to decrease. Watch the monitors carefully, use occasional big breaths among lots of tidal volume breaths. This has the potential to offer effective treatment without compromising BP. It is vital to watch the bedside monitors during manual hyperinflation to monitor the patient's cardiovascular response.

CASE STUDY 2 – PAEDIATRIC INTENSIVE CARE UNIT

Elaine Dhouieb

A 2-year-old girl, previously well, with normal birth and no past medical history of note, was admitted to ICU 3 days previously with bacterial tracheitis. Unwell at home 1 day, had cold and corzal signs 2 days.

On Examination

Intubated nasally; paralysed and sedated; i.v. antibiotics; tube feeds NG; no inotropes.

Now cardiovascularly stable, no deterioration with handling.

Heart rate 120 BP 100/50 CVP 10

Heart rate increases with handling

SpO$_2$ had been steady at around 95% – now 90%

On antibiotics; paralysis; sedation; hourly NG feeds

Pressure controlled ventilation RR 20 b.p.m.

Pressure increased to 25 over 6 as PaCO$_2$ increased on last gas (6 kPa)

Oxygen increased from 40% to 60% because of saturations and decreased PaO$_2$ on last gas (8 kPa); slightly acidotic (pH 7.2)

Has had moderate mucopurulent secretions and started chest physiotherapy today

CXR this evening shows right upper lobe collapse

In supine, decreased expansion on right side visible from examination

Auscultation: Bronchial breathing right upper lobe

More secretions with physiotherapy than with nurses bagging and suctioning

Copious nasal discharge

Questions:
1 How do you communicate with the parents?
2 What can you discuss with the nurses to assist in keeping the patient stable during treatment?
3 What would your physiotherapy treatment plan be?

Answer 1:

- Introduce yourself, explain to her parents the need for treatment and the procedure. Mother decides to stay, father prefers to leave. Physiotherapy can be worrying for parents with no experience of respiratory physiotherapy.

Answer 2:

- Give an extra bolus of sedation to prevent distress – she is obviously aware as her heart rate increases with handling. She may have swelling of her airway and it is important that she does not move. Check with the nurses that the paralysing agent is adequate.
- Check how secure tube is as she has copious nasal discharge and it may need to be retaped before treatment.

Answer 3:

- MHI by nurse. Quick expiration to move secretions.
- Percussion and vibrations in supine. (Position for RUL, percussion to loosen secretions, vibrations to move up bronchial tree.)
- Suction. Thick mucopurulent secretions.
- Assess stability, air entry and chest movement.
- Repeat if necessary.
- Tolerated treatment well. Good air entry and good chest movement. SpO_2 up to 98% back on ventilator.
- Advise nurses that there is no need to be nursed supine (move to prevent accumulation of secretions in one position, patient stable enough to be turned).
- Assist in gentle turn, taking account of line positions. Support in half side-lying with support for limbs.
- Leave to rest, staff to repeat gases in 30 minutes and reassess ventilation.

CASE STUDY 3 – MEDICAL UNIT

Sarah Keilty

A 70-year-old woman with pneumonia. Admitted via A&E via GP with chest pain and increased SOB. Two-day history of productive cough with yellow sputum, vomiting.

History

PMH: Ischaemic heart disease

10.00 hours
ABGs in A&E FiO_2 0.35
pH 7.320 $PaCO_2$ 3.1 PaO_2 9.2
BE -1.9 HCO_3^- 25
Observations:
Temperature 38.1 Heart rate 80
BP 120/70 RR 28 SpO_2 95%
Blood tests: WCC 17.3 Normal chemistry
CXR shows R LL pneumonia
Auscultation: Bronchial breathing R base

Seen on the ward round. Plan: commenced on i.v. antibiotics and 35% oxygen therapy. Commence i.v. fluids as patient not taking oral fluids.

13.00 h House Officer (HO) called to review patient as patient condition deteriorating with increased SOB and chest pain.
Observations:
Temperature 37.1 HR 120 atrial fibrillation (AF)
BP 130/70 RR 28 SpO_2 85%
Dry, unproductive cough.
Physiotherapist asked to review patient.

Question:

1 What physiotherapy treatment would be appropriate?

Then …
16.00 h S/B medical team – continue on antibiotics and start digoxin to treat AF.

Observations:
Temperature 37.5 HR 120 BP 140/80
RR 30 SpO_2 96% on 60% O_2

19.30 h HO on call asked to review patient.
Patient looks more SOB, with SpO_2 at 90% and HR 135 (AF).
Coarse crackles heard on auscultation. Registrar reviews patient and calls on call physiotherapist.

Question:
2 What would you ask for to help make an accurate assessment and what other things could be done while you are on your way in?

Then …
20.00 h Physiotherapy review
Observations:
Temperature 37.6 HR 115 BP 140/60
RR 35 SpO_2 92% on 60% oxygen
WCC 16

ABGs pH 7.44 $PaCO_2$ 3.74
          PaO_2 9.0 HCO_3^- 25
          BE −1.2 Lactate 1.5
Coarse crackles heard on auscultation. Ineffective cough, unable to clear secretions.
Patient tells you she is too tired to cough any more.

Question:
3 What treatment could you do to facilitate mucus expectoration and improve oxygenation?

Then …
Post treatment; SpO_2 increases to 95% on 60%
Physiotherapist suggests increased oxygen delivery (e.g. rebreathe bag) or CPAP if patient becomes more hypoxic.

22.30 hours HO returns to review patient. Patient exhausted, with rapid shallow breathing pattern. Repeat blood gases.

ABGs 23.00
          FiO_2 0.6 pH 7.32 PCO_2 7.0
          PO_2 10.3 HCO_3^- 23 BE −1.3
(Patient has not had CPAP)

The patient has a respiratory acidosis. HO on call concerned as she is elderly and in view of high PaO_2 but rise in CO_2, and feels that the patient may have oxygen induced CO_2 retention. FiO_2 reduced by HO to 28%.

Question:
4 Did the doctor interpret the gases correctly?

Then ...

Physiotherapist called again. Correct interpretation of blood gases means that oxygen can be increased to maintain $SpO_2 > 90\%$. Thus FiO_2 increased back up to 60% following discussion with medical team. Secretions cleared with IPPB as suggested in answer 4, but it is clear that this patient is going to require some assistance with her breathing.

Question:
5 What would .be the best mode of respiratory support?

Answer 1:
• Positioned in to left side-lying to try and improve ventilation–perfusion and thus reduce the work of breathing. In discussion with the doctor increased FiO_2 to 0.6, as she is extremely hypoxic. As she has high flow oxygen and retained secretions it is appropriate to advise humidification.

Answer 2:
• Arterial blood gases, repeat CXR and saline nebulizers. Does the patient need any salbutamol?

Answer 3:
• Treatment. Positioned on to left side-lying, IPPB (as unable to take big breath) with chest shaking on expiration. Followed by some breathing control, forced expiration technique ('huffing'). Patient able to cough and expectorate sputum.

Answer 4:
• The patient has a respiratory acidosis (raised CO_2 with reduced pH). However, the cause was wrongly interpreted. The patient has

developed ventilatory failure, and a respiratory acidosis secondary to her severe increased work of breathing and respiratory muscle fatigue. The HCO_3 is within normal limits and thus this patient does not have acute on chronic CO_2 retention. Thus it is safe to give the patient as much O_2 as she requires.

Answer 5:
- NIV plus supplemental oxygen overnight would be ideal, with anaesthetic review if NIV is not able to correct her acid–base balance. If you do not have access to NIV, anaesthetic review would be needed and the decision made whether to intubate and ventilate the patient.

CASE STUDY 4 – SURGICAL UNIT

Valerie Ball
Call to a 52-year-old woman, current smoker.
Elective total abdominal hysterectomy 2 days ago.
Increasing shortness of breath over a period of 12 h.
Not previously referred to ward physiotherapist.

History
PMH: Occasional asthma

Medical Management Since Deterioration
Morphine (PCA), O_2, antibiotics, digoxin
ABGs taken on 60% O_2

> pH 7.43 $PaCO_2$ 4.8
> PaO_2 7.6 HCO_3^- 25.4

Chest X-ray ordered – shows total left lung opacity with raised hemidiaphragm.

Patient transferred to high dependency unit.
Physiotherapist called.

Question:
1 What would you ask to be done while en route to the ward?

On Examination

Subjective examination:
Distressed but cooperative, clammy to touch.
Afraid to take a deep breath or cough, but feels the need to cough.
Objective examination:
Sat upright in bed
Mildly obese lady
Temperature 38.9°C Heart rate 140/min
Blood pressure 111/75 Respiratory rate 35/min
Left side chest movement decreased

SpO$_2$ 89% on O$_2$ driven nebulizer (Ventolin) Humidifier warming up
Auscultation: Normal breath sounds right side of chest, bronchial breathing entire left side of chest.
Urine output inconclusive, no hourly measurement prior to HDU transfer.

Problem

Profound volume loss left lung causing acute hypoxaemia.

Questions:
2 What treatment techniques would you employ?
3 What precautions would you take?

Answer 1:

- The patient has a collapsed lung probably due to sputum plugging. Contributory factors include:
  a. smoking history
  b. asthma
  c. recent anaesthesia.
- Request that patient's pain relief is optimized.
- Ask for a humidifier to be set up with high flow O$_2$ (if available, otherwise it may only be possible to temporarily administer a higher percentage of dry oxygen or humidified CPAP) as the patient is receiving 60% oxygen but is still hypoxaemic.

Answer 2:

- Reassure patient; explain what you want her to do and how to use the PCA to help.

279

- Position in right side-lying to:
  a. improve V/Q matching
  b. drain the left lung.
- Teach the patient how to perform an active cycle of breathing, FET and supported coughing. Continue with cycles with consideration for pain relief and avoiding fatigue until no further secretions can be expectorated.
- Reassess:
  a. respiratory rate – is it falling? is the patient tiring? Check $PaCO_2$.
  b. SaO_2 – is it rising?
  c. breath sounds at regular intervals – are normal breath sounds appearing?
- Consider progressing to postural drainage positions, using Flutter valve, or IPPB.

Answer 3:

- Monitor heart rate and blood pressure. A heart rate of 140/min is a relative contraindication to physiotherapy. The reasons for treating outweigh the precautions because:
  a. there is no history of heart disease
  b. high heart rate is likely to be result of intrapulmonary shunt caused by large unventilated area of lung.
- If the heart rate rises or the blood pressure falls outside of patient's normal limits, the medical team must be informed and a decision made about continuing further.
- Monitor carefully for bronchospasm (asthma history). Ask the patient if she can detect symptoms and/or use auscultation to detect expiratory wheeze. Gentle rhythmic percussion is tolerated by some patients and may be added into the active cycle to increase clearance rate.

CASE STUDY 5 – NEUROLOGICAL UNIT

Lorraine Clapham

Call to see a 52-year-old man admitted with progressive muscle weakness affecting all four limbs.

History

PMH: No previous hospital admissions, minor illnesses only
SH: Married, schoolteacher. Non-smoker usually very active

Medical Findings on Admission

Alert, orientated

Cranial nerves – intact

Motor power – proximal muscle weakness grade 3–4

Sensation – intact

Respiratory system:

Trachea central Respiratory rate 20

Normal breath sounds Vital capacity 5 litres

CXR – elevated right hemidiaphragm

ABGs:

$$\text{pH } 7.4 \quad PaCO_2 \text{ } 4.49 \quad PaO_2 \text{ } 9.9$$
$$HCO_3^- \text{ } 22 \quad O_2 \text{ Saturation } 95\% \text{ on air}$$

Provisional diagnosis – Guillain–Barré Syndrome

Call for physiotherapy – 6 hours after admission

Reason given for call out – vital capacity has fallen to 1.6 L, now requiring 35% oxygen and is maintaining oxygen saturation levels at 96%

Questions:

1 Given that oxygen saturation levels are being maintained at 96% on FiO_2 of 35%, from the information provided, what indications are there for emergency on call physiotherapy?

2 What further information will you require, and what will be the key elements of your assessment?

3 At this stage, what are your treatment options (management plan)?

Answer 1:

- There has been a rapid and major deterioration in the patient's condition. Vital capacity has fallen by almost a quarter. The patient's ability to take a sigh breath is impaired, as is his ability to clear any retained secretions. Some degree of atelectasis will have already occurred. This will probably progress to major lobar collapse and sputum retention.

- On admission there were already signs that would have predicted the possibility of respiratory deterioration:

   a. The elevated right diaphragm in the absence of obvious lobar collapse suggests that there is some degree of paralysis of this muscle.

b. The high respiratory rate and low CO_2 suggest that the patient is working very hard to maintain his PaO_2 and oxygen saturation levels at 96%.

- Without intervention this patient is likely to fatigue quickly and progress to respiratory failure and require ventilation.

Answer 2:

- Observe and assess the patient.
- Arterial blood gases are essential; the patient may already be retaining CO_2.
- Repeat chest X-ray.
- Is there any indication that the patient may be at risk of aspiration, e.g. wet sounding voice, reports of coughing when drinking?

Answer 3:

- Position the patient so as to reduce the work of breathing (see Ch. 7).
- Humidify oxygen.
- Reassure the patient.
- IPPB to inflate lung and improve lung compliance thus reduce the work of breathing and oxygen demand.
- Patient review in 1 h, repeat vital capacity and ABGs.
- If CO_2 continues to rise ventilation will need to be discussed. Depending on the team decision this may be NIV, if available, or full ventilation. Care must be taken not to mask a deteriorating patient – close monitoring is essential.
- Review as planned.
- Inform staff of current action plan and leave contact number.
- If patient's condition stabilizes or improves, continue with current treatment plan and monitoring.
- Ensure intensive care has been alerted to the problem. If the patient continues to deteriorate a planned intubation is preferable to an emergency intubation.

CASE STUDY 6 – CARDIOTHORACIC UNIT

Sarah Boyce

A 58-year-old man, CABG × 5, 2 days ago. The doctor has called you in because the patient has become 'chesty'. On further questioning you discover that they have ordered a chest X-ray.

Observations:
BP 95/50 HR 120 Urine output has decreased throughout the day
SaO_2 92% FiO_2 0.6 RR of 26

Questions:
1 What could be the possible causes of the low blood pressure and how could this be stabilized for treatment?
2 What could be making the patient 'chesty'?
3 What physiotherapy treatments may be appropriate?

Answer 1:

Potential cause	Treatment
Hypovolaemia	Fluid replacement. If active bleeding point will require surgical intervention
Cardiac failure	Inotropic support, e.g. noradrenaline (norepinephrine), adrenaline (epinephrine) or dopamine
Arrhythmia (typically AF)	This can compromise BP, usually treated with digoxin, or in severe cases the patient may be cardioverted

Answers 2 and 3:

Cause	Treatment
Sputum retention could be related to pain, infection or anxiety. Also consider may be very heavy smoker, five grafts shows extensive damage. Look for signs of infection	Optimize analgesia. Positioning (mobilization not advised) unless BP improved. Humidification. TEEs or ACBT with inspiratory hold and sniff, with encouragement. IPPB if unable to take effective deep breath
Pulmonary oedema	CPAP very effective means of maintaining oxygenation while waiting for medical treatment, e.g. furosemide (frusemide) to work
Could be a mixture of sputum retention and pulmonary oedema	As above may consider using both IPPB and CPAP if necessary

283

CASE STUDY 7 – ONCOLOGY UNIT

Katharine Malhotra and Nicola Thompson

A 28-year-old man with acute myeloid leukaemia (AML), 8 days post induction chemotherapy.

History
PMH: No previous hospital admissions.
SH: Single. Sales rep. Non-smoker. Hobbies: running; mountain biking; swimming.

Medical Management
Blood counts
WCC 0.2 Platelets 22 Hb 9.3
Temperature 38.5 Blood pressure 100/55
SaO_2 91% Fluids in progress
CXR ordered – diffuse changes both lung fields, no local consolidation or collapse
Provisional diagnosis – chest infection

Call Out
Deteriorating respiratory function with X-ray changes. On call physiotherapist asked to review. Doctors requesting a sputum specimen to isolate cause.

Subjective Examination

Patient frightened because unable to breathe

Feeling shivery and cold

Questions:
1 What further information will you require and what will be the key elements of your assessment?
2 At this stage what are your treatment options?
3 What would you document in the medical notes?

Answer 1:
Need to look at:

Bone Marrow Function
(has recent chemotherapy suppressed the bone marrow?)

- Blood counts.
- WCC – low white cell count would suggest low sputum production and atypical infection.
- Platelet count – a low count would modify the treatment technique chosen.
- If the patient has had a platelet transfusion recently.
- If there are any signs of active bleeding – if so treatment would need to be done during or after platelet transfusion.

Respiratory Function
(might this patient be progressing towards respiratory failure?)

- How long has the patient had respiratory symptoms and have they ever been productive?
- Arterial blood gas results to give indication of ventilation gas exchange and acid–base status. Just how hypoxic are they?
- Respiratory rate currently and as a trend – how quickly is the rate changing with what inspired oxygen concentration?
- Look at pattern/distribution of CXR changes. Is there bilateral hilar shadowing with clear apex and bases to indicate *Pneumocystis carinii* pneumonia (PCP)?

Cardiac Function
(might this patient be progressing towards septic shock?)

- Recent blood pressure reading to highlight any cardiovascular instability.
- Are the fluids being given to support cardiac output or are they intravenous antibiotics for the chest?
- How are the heart rate and blood pressure behaving in relation to the fever and respiratory rate?

Objective Examination Would Include
- Observation of posture, mental status, respiratory rate, breathing pattern, colour of patient.
- Auscultation to determine presence of breath sounds and added sounds.

Answer 2:
Sputum clearance techniques not indicated because of:

- lack of evidence for sputum being present
- bruising/bleeding risk with low platelets
- unnecessary challenge to stressed respiratory and cardiac systems.

Consider work of breathing:

- Is oxygen prescription appropriate both in amount and method of delivery?
- Is position assisting respiratory muscle effort?
- Does the patient understand why small efforts (talking/eating/turning in bed) make him feel so breathless?

Answer 3:

- At this stage physiotherapy treatment is limited and it is unlikely that a sputum specimen will be obtainable. If the doctors are waiting for a specimen before treating the chest infection they may want to initiate drug therapy presumptively rather than wait.
- The patient's main problem is increased work of breathing associated with hypoxia, pyrexia, cardiovascular instability.
- Positioning can help but if the patient continues to deteriorate in his respiratory rate despite increasing inspired oxygen then an anaesthetic opinion is likely to be more helpful than physiotherapy.

NOTE: There are differences in the way PCP presents in haematology oncology and HIV disease:

- In HIV the onset is slower with more erosive changes to the lung tissue forming bullae and creating the risk of spontaneous pneumothorax. Bone marrow suppression is not a feature. The problems remain primarily problems of ventilation.
- In haematology oncology the immunosuppression is more profound producing a more rapid development of symptoms, more systemic sepsis and greater risk of shock. Bone marrow suppression is an important factor in treatment selection. In the critically ill, the problems may be perfusion as much as ventilation related.

CASE STUDY 8 – NEONATAL UNIT

Allie Carter

A 26-week preterm infant, now 30 weeks, corrected with chronic lung disease.

Ventilated since birth.

Has on several occasions needed high frequency oscillatory ventilation. Copious secretions requiring regular suction.

Has cleared secretions mainly with suction but needing intermittent physiotherapy.

HPC: Multiple areas of collapse – right and left upper lobes

Retention of secretions

Climbing CO_2

Now on nitric oxide

Due to instability nursed only in supine with head only being turned

Questions:
1 What are the main problems?
2 What precautions would you consider prior to treatment?
3 What modifications would you make to the treatment?
4 What advice would you make for ongoing care?

Answer 1:
Main Problems:
- Are you trained adequately to treat a neonate? If not, don't
- High oxygen requirement
- Ventilated on high O_2
- High pressures
- Thick secretions
- Difficult to clear sputum with infant in supine due to instability
- Decreased breath sounds
- CXR – severe collapse
- Clinical evidence of severe secretion retention.

Answer 2:
Precautions:
- Osteopenia
- Changes of position not tolerated
- Check abdomen and cerebral state.

Answer 3:
Treatment Modifications:
- Always have a nurse to assist
- Position changes even by 45 degrees

- Use of active techniques
- Saline with treatment and suction
- Closed suction circuit
- Preoxygenation.

Answer 4:
Advice for Ongoing Care:
- 4 hourly turns for next 4–6 h, with 4–6 hourly physiotherapy
- Use of quarter turns but prone included if possible
- Use of more saline if necessary
- Assess and reassess
- Continue prophylactic positioning regime.

Results:
- Infant received physiotherapy and regular turns overnight.
- Ventilation reduced.
- Secretions gradually cleared.
- NO removed within 24 h.
- Gases improved considerably.

CASE STUDY 9 – PAEDIATRIC WARD

Paul Ritson
You are called to the paediatric medical ward to see a 15-month-old girl who has been admitted from casualty 2 h ago with a severe chest infection.

On the telephone, you are given the following information:

1 2-day history of productive cough
2 Apnoeic episodes last hour on ward, responding to stimulation
3 SpO_2 90% in 6 litres per minute via nasal cannulae
4 Suction required frequently, yielding copious thick green secretions
5 Arterial blood gas, pH 7.29, $PaCO_2$ 75 mmHg (10 kPa), PaO_2 60 mmHg (8 kPa), base excess +1
6 Chest X-ray (Fig. 19.1) taken 10 minutes ago, not yet seen by doctor.

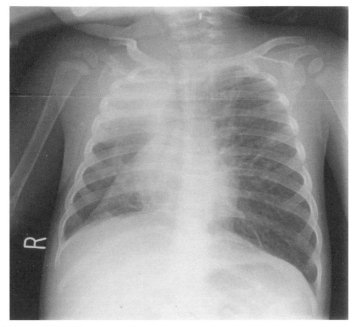

Figure 19.1   X-ray in paediatric case study 9.

Questions:
1   What further information do you require over the telephone, and what advice could you give, to be carried out before your arrival on the ward?
2   On arrival, how would you plan your assessment?
3   Look at the CXR and the blood gas result. What do they show?
4   Devise a possible treatment plan for this patient.

Answer 1:
Information Required:
- How is the child responding to handling?
- Obtain more clinical details, e.g. neurological/CVS.
- What position is the patient in?
- How often is suction being carried out?

- OP or NP suction?
- Are any nebulizers needed; if so, which ones?
- Any pre-existing pathologies that may affect respiratory status?

Answer 2:
Advice Given:
- Change O_2 delivery from nasal cannulae to humidified O_2 via head box or face mask if tolerated.
- Change patient position to side-lying with 'head up' position, well supported with pillow/towel/teddy.
- Give bronchodilator (if prescribed) before arrival or give saline nebulizers to loosen secretions.
- Increase FiO_2 via head box to keep SpO_2 above 95%.

Answer 3:
Plan Assessment:
- Be methodical
- Full subjective assessment
- Full objective assessment
- Problem list
- Treatment plan
- Use Chapters 3 and 17.

CXR:
- Mediastinal shift to right
- Elevated right hemidiaphragm
- Hyperinflated left lung
- Partial right lower lobe collapse
- Right upper lobe collapse
- Nasogastric tube in stomach.

Blood Gas Analysis:
- Hypoxia $PO_2 < 80$ mmHg (10.7 kPa)
- Hypercapnic $PCO_2 > 45$ mmHg (6.0 kPa)
- Acidotic pH < 7.35
- Normal base
- Uncompensated respiratory acidosis.

Answer 4:
Treatment Plan:
- Explanation to parents/carers about consent to treatment and treatment plan.

- Positioning: probably left side-lying with 'head up', to treat right upper lobe.
- Positioning: probably left side lying flat or head down to treat right lower lobe (care with head down tipping).
- Assess SpO_2 in this position, change position if necessary (be aware of ventilation/perfusion differences in paediatrics).
- Humidification via head box – heated if bronchospasm is evident (use a temperature probe to prevent burns).
- Manual techniques as indicated.
- Nasopharyngeal suction if indicated.
- Bronchodilators if indicated.
- Frequent position changes if tolerating handling, keeping 'head up' position (2–3 hourly).
- Regular reassessment.
- Discussion with nursing staff about assessment findings and plan for further management.

CHAPTER 20

Reflection upon the call out experience

Jane Cross

Many physiotherapists who work on call feel uncertain whether they possess the skills and attributes required for this high-speed, complex environment. This service, like any other in the health service today, is subject to quality measures and standards. The clinical governance concept outlined in *The New NHS: Modern and Dependable* (DoH 1997) has made it clear that quality exists not only as a responsibility of the organization but also for each professional working in it. This agenda may well have exacerbated individuals' feelings of vulnerability and decreased their confidence.

The intention of this chapter is to provide you with insight into some of the ways in which you can assess your own learning needs, prepare for being on call and learn from each on call episode. During the chapter a number of tools that can facilitate you in this process will be referred to. The reporting of these is necessarily brief and will not deal in any detail with any of the particular tools suggested. Reference will be made to other work which develops these ideas further and should be used as a reading list for you when you are developing and demonstrating your competency in the on call setting. Start by contacting your professional body to obtain the latest information on standards for on call working. This will guide you through the process.

HOW CAN WE PREPARE FOR AN ON CALL EVENT?

Reflect:

* What do you know already?
* What do you need to know?

Spend a moment thinking about what you already know and what you need to know. Reflection is about learning from experience (Spalding 1998) and as such is a valuable tool for the practitioner from the perspective of their own professional development.

Reflection:
Further reading which is presented as a personal experience of using reflection to demonstrate professional development can be found in Spalding (1998).

- Complete a SWOT analysis.

SWOT Analysis:
Tools such as a SWOT analysis (strengths, weaknesses, opportunities and threats) can be useful in this process. For further information and an illustration of the use of this tool see Atkinson (1998).

The process of producing a SWOT analysis can be undertaken as a piece of individual reflection. However, it could also be facilitated by a peer. Ask someone to help you. A colleague could help you recognize some of the strengths, weaknesses, etc. that you have in relation to working on call.

Once you are clear upon what your needs are and recognize some of your strengths, it may be useful to set up a learning contract with yourself and/or your manager or senior member of staff, as appropriate. Alternatively add these needs to your existing personal development plan (PDP).

Learning Contracts:
This contract should identify the means by which an individual can achieve their identified learning needs. These means could include work experience opportunities, teaching sessions that they would like to attend, internally organized training programmes as well as external courses and perhaps more formal routes of academic learning. This list is by no means exhaustive. Individuals and their managers should be as innovative as possible when trying to identify the means of meeting these learning needs. The more formalized external routes of leaning should only be contemplated when internal resources cannot meet these needs. Included within the contract should be review dates and evaluative measures. For more information regarding learning contracts see Walker (1999).

- Arrange for an induction.

Talk to those who work in the areas you are likely to be called into. Arrange to spend some time with them. You may need a guided tour of where equipment is kept, or a quick talk through some of the processes operated on individual wards. Spend some time on the intensive care unit (ICU) and high dependency unit (HDU) so that you can see the equipment in use and meet some of the staff who work there.

Try to meet some of these needs before your first on call event but recognize some of these will take longer to fulfil than others!

HOW CAN WE LEARN FROM THE ON CALL EVENT?

- Recording your thoughts following your on call, either as a critical incident or as part of your reflective diary, will form a useful record of your thoughts and feelings at this time. This record will help you recognize your learning needs for the future but also, and possibly more importantly, it will help you recognize the progress you are making in your efforts to enhance your competence.
- Follow your on call event up with a 'debrief' either as a paper exercise for yourself or with a colleague or the senior member of staff with responsibility for on call.

Ask:
- How did it go?
- What went well?
- What could have gone better?
- Why do you think that particular aspect went well/not so well?
- How could you improve upon that aspect?
- What do you need to do in order to improve that aspect?
- How can that be facilitated?
- Do you need any resources in order to achieve this?

Answering these questions, may help you to reflect upon your experience and identify what you have learned and what further learning you need to undertake to achieve the enhanced competence that you seek.

If you choose to 'debrief' with another person certain criteria need to be met to ensure that this is a learning event. The person with whom you undertake this debriefing/reflection must be able to support you in a non-threatening way. Their role is to facilitate you in your thinking about your clinical reasoning and your resulting actions. They need to help you identify what went well and what could have been improved. By doing this you can then identify ongoing learning needs and identify ways in which these can be achieved.

- Use your learning diary to facilitate this period of reflection with another therapist.
- Use your learning diary to facilitate your own individual and internalized reflective activity.

Learning Diary/Learning Log:
The use of a learning diary, in which a clinician records on call situations, their actions, the clinical reasoning which led to these actions and their feelings about the situation, could be used as a record from which an individual could demonstrate their competency. It could actually be referred to as written down reflection. Furthermore it can be used as a useful learning tool. For example, if excerpts from this were used during a debriefing (reflection), following an on call episode, this process could be turned into a learning event.

Critical Incident Report (this is within the context of learning, not risk management!):
Incidents such as these occur throughout our working lives. They do not have to be awful moments, they can be really positive moments when we know we have done something really well. Alternatively they could be 'ah ha' moments, such as when the penny drops when battling to understand a difficult concept or skill that we have been grappling with for a while. Recording these moments can help us identify how and what we have learned from a given situation or moment. Recording these can help us later, as a record of what it was we felt we had achieved. They can also facilitate our 'reflection on action' (Schon 1991) which is the term coined for thinking about an incident some time after it has occurred to identify what went well/wrong so that we can learn more from it and thus move on further in our learning process.

- Include a critical incident analysis in your learning diary.

HOW CAN WE DEMONSTRATE WHAT WE HAVE LEARNED?

Use the tools we have identified to create a portfolio which can be used to demonstrate the progress you have made.

Portfolio:

This is a collection of material that we can present to demonstrate to others that we have achieved the learning that we set out to do. This planned learning can be evidenced by including, in a portfolio, SWOT analyses and learning contracts. Evidence that this learning has been achieved could include extracts from learning diaries/logs, critical incident reports, anonymous case study reports, extracts from courses, training sessions attended, etc. It is important, however, with this type of collection of evidence that the individual remembers that they will be bringing this into the public arena. Particular attention should thus be paid to maintaining the confidentiality both of others – professional and patient – and of ourselves. Further reading can be found in Stewart (1998).

- Participate in some case studies where you can use real or imaginary cases to demonstrate your clinical reasoning. You could also use these in preparation for on call to practice your clinical reasoning.

Case Studies:

Sound clinical reasoning is one such skill and is essential for safe practice across the spectrum of physiotherapy work. This is one of the hardest areas to assess regarding the competency issue. Using case studies in on call/respiratory in service education is one way in which clinicians can assess competency in this area. Real or imaginary case studies can be used to examine the clinical reasoning process in a variety of settings and covering a variety of topics. Both the educator and the learner can take responsibility for producing these and they can be used as a record for an individual's portfolio. Examples of such studies can be found in Chapter 19 of this book. For further reading about using clinical reasoning as a tool for demonstrating continuing professional development see Stephenson (1998).

- Undertake peer review with a colleague. You could choose to work on a case together or use incidents from your learning diary or a critical incident.
- Link closely with your mentor to develop your learning.

Peer Review:
This is another method by which the clinician can assess their own and others' competency. This tool could be used both in the here and now by treating a real patient and going through the reasoning with a colleague who is present both during the treatment and afterwards. Incidents from your learning log or critical incident reports could also be the stimulus for discussion. This can follow on from the use of case studies as outlined earlier.

Ground rules need to be established and agreed before these sessions take place and these should include how an individual would like to receive feedback, the confidentiality that is to be expected both on the part of the reviewed and the reviewer and what type of record of the session is to be kept.

Following the ideas in this chapter can help you prepare well for your first on call event, plan your learning and record your achievements. This should help you as adult learners take responsibility for your own learning and empower you to ask for the support that you need to achieve both confidence and competence in an on call situation.

References

Atkinson K (1998) SWOT analysis: a tool for continuing professional development. BJTR 5(8):433–435.

Department of Health (1997) White Paper. The New NHS: Modern, Dependable. London: HMSO.

Schon D (1991) The reflective practitioner: how professionals think in action, 2nd edn. San Francisco: Jossey Bass.

Spalding N (1998) Reflection in professional development: a personal experience. BJTR 5(7):379–382.

Stephenson R (1998) Can clinical reasoning be an effective tool in CPD? BJTR 5(6):325–329.

Stewart S (1998) The place of portfolios in continuing professional development. BJTR 5(5):266–269.

Walker E (1999) Learning contracts in practice: their role in CPD. BJTR 6(2):91–94.

APPENDICES

Appendix 1

NORMAL VALUES

Table to show normal values. Reproduced with kind permission of Pryor and Prasad (2002).

Normal Values

Age group	Heart rate Mean (range) (beats/min)	Respiratory rate range (breaths/min)	Blood pressure systolic/diastolic (mmHg)
Preterm	150 (100–200)	40–60	39–59 / 16–36
Newborn	140 (80–200)	30–50	50–70 / 25–45
<2 years	130 (100–190)	20–40	87–105 / 53–66
>2 years	80 (60–140)	20–40	95–105 /53–66
>6 years	75 (60–90)	15–30	97–112 / 57–71
Adults	70 (50–100)	12–16	95–140 / 60–90

Conversion Tables

0.133 kPa = 1.0 mmHg		$pH = 9 - \log[H^+]$ where $[H^+]$ is in nmol/l	
kPa	mmHg	pH	$[H^+]$
1	7.5	7.52	30
2	15.0	7.45	35
4	30	7.40	40
6	45	7.35	45
8	60	7.30	50
10	75	7.26	55
12	90	7.22	60
14	105	7.19	65

Arterial Blood

pH	7.35–7.45 [H^+] 45–35 nmol/L
PaO_2	10.7–13.3 kPa (80–100 mmHg)
$PaCO_2$	4.7–6.0 kPa (35–45 mmHg)
HCO_3^-	22–26 mmol/L
Base excess	-2 to $+2$

Venous Blood

pH	7.31–7.41 [H^+] 46–38 nmol/L
PO_2	5.0–5.6 kPa (37–42 mmHg)
PCO_2	5.6–6.7 kPa (42–50 mmHg)

Ventilation/Perfusion

Alveolar–arterial oxygen gradient A–aPO_2:

Breathing air	0.7–2.7 kPa (5–20 mmHg)
Breathing 100% oxygen	3.3–8.6 kPa (25–65 mmHg)

Pressures

		mmHg	kPa
Right atrial (RA) pressure	Mean	-1 to $+7$	-0.13 to 0.93
Right ventricular (RV) pressure	Systolic	15–25	2.0–3.3
	Diastolic	0–8	0–1.0
Pulmonary artery (PA) pressure	Systolic	15–25	2.0–3.3
	Diastolic	8–15	1.0–2.0
	Mean	10–20	1.3–2.7
Pulmonary capillary wedge pressure (PCWP)	Mean	6–15	0.8–2.0
Central venous pressure (CVP)		3–15 cmH_2O	
Intracranial pressure (ICP)		<10 mmHg (<1.3 kPa)	
Peak inspiratory mouth pressure (PiMax)	Male	103–124 cmH_2O (age dependent)	
	Female	65–87 cmH_2O (age dependent)	
Peak expiratory mouth pressure (PeMax)	Male	185–233 cmH_2O (age dependent)	
	Female	128–152 cmH_2O (age dependent)	

Blood Chemistry

Albumin	37–53 g/L
Calcium (Ca^{2+})	2.25–2.65 mmol/L
Creatinine	60–120 µmol/L
Glucose	4–6 mmol/L
Potassium (K^+)	3.4–5.0 mmol/L
Sodium (Na^+)	134–140 mmol/L
Urea	2.5–6.5 mmol/L
Haemoglobin (Hb)	14.0–18.0 g/100 ml (men)
	11.5–15.5 g/100 ml (women)
Platelets	150–400 $\times 10^9$/L
White blood cell count (WBC)	4–11 $\times 10^9$/L
Urine output	1 ml/kg/h

Appendix 2

COMMON SURGICAL INCISIONS

Figure showing (**A** and **B**) common surgical incisions. Reproduced with kind permission of Pryor and Prasad (2002).

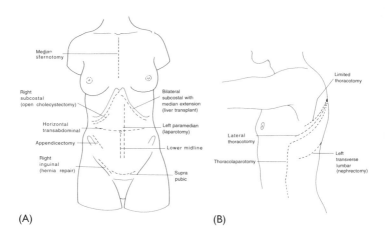

Appendix 3

ABBREVIATIONS

A&E	Accident & Emergency
ABG	arterial blood gas
ACBT	active cycle of breathing techniques
ACPRC	Association of Chartered Physiotherapists in Respiratory Care
AD	autogenic drainage
AF	atrial fibrillation
ALI	acute lung injury
AML	acute myeloid leukaemia
AP	anteroposterior
ARDS	acute respiratory distress syndrome
ASD	atrial septal defect
Ausc.	auscultation
AVSD	atrioventricular septal defect
AVR	aortic valve replacement
BAL	bronchoalveolar lavage
BC	breathing control
BE	base excess
BOS	base of skull
BP	blood pressure (arterial)
BPD	bronchopulmonary dysplasia
b.p.m.	beats per minute
BS	breath sounds
CABG	coronary artery bypass graft
CCF	congestive cardiac failure
CF	cystic fibrosis
CFM	cerebral function monitor
CMD	congenital muscular dystrophy

CMV	continuous mandatory ventilation
CMV	cytomegalovirus
CNS	central nervous system
CO_2	carbon dioxide
COAD	chronic obstructive airways disease
COPD	chronic obstructive pulmonary disease
CP	cerebral palsy
CPAP	continuous positive airways pressure
CPP	cerebral perfusion pressure
CSF	cerebrospinal fluid
CSP	Chartered Society of Physiotherapy
CVA	cerebrovascular accident
CVP	central venous pressure
CVS	cardiovascular system
CXR	Chest X-ray
DH	drug history
DIC	disseminated intravascular coagulation
DMD	Duchenne muscular dystrophy
DVT	deep vein thrombosis
ECG	electrocardiogram
ECMO	extracorporeal membrane oxygenation
ENT	Ear Nose & Throat
ETT	endotracheal tube
EVD	external ventricular drain
Fen.	fenestrated
FET	forced expiration technique
FEV_1	forced vital capacity in first second of expiration
FiO_2	fraction of inspired oxygen
FRC	functional residual capacity
FVC	forced vital capacity
GAP	gravity assisted positioning
GCS	Glasgow Coma Scale
GI	gastrointestinal
GOR	gastro-oesophageal reflux
Hb	haemoglobin
HCO_3^-	bicarbonate ions

HDU	high dependency unit
HF	haemofiltration
HFO	high frequency oscillation
HPC	history of present condition
HR	heart rate
IABP	intra-aortic balloon pump
ICD	intercostal drain
ICP	intracranial pressure
ICU	intensive care unit
IHD	ischaemic heart disease
i.m.	intramuscular
INR	international clotting ratio
IPPB	intermittent positive pressure breathing
IS	incentive spirometry
i.v.	intravenous
JVP	jugular venous pressure
K^+	potassium ions
LFT	lung function test *or* liver function test
LLL	left lower lobe
LTOT	long-term oxygen therapy
LUL	left upper lobe
LVF	left ventricular failure
LZ	lower zone
MAP	mean arterial pressure
MHI	manual hyperinflation
MT	manual techniques
MV	minute volume
MVR	mitral valve replacement
MZ	middle zone
Na^+	sodium ions
NaCl	sodium chloride
NAI	non-accidental injury
NBM	nil by mouth
NCA	nurse controlled analgesia

NGT	nasogastric tube
NIV	non-invasive ventilation
NO	nitric oxide
NP	nasopharangeal
NSAIDs	non-steroidal anti-inflammatory drugs

O_2	oxygen
OP	oropharyngeal

PA	posteroanterior
$PaCO_2$	partial pressure of carbon dioxide in arterial blood
PaO_2	partial pressure of oxygen in arterial blood
PAP	peak airway pressure
PAWP	pulmonary artery wedge pressure
PCA	patient controlled analgesia
PCEA	patient controlled epidural anaesthesia
PCP	*Pneumocystis carinii* pneumonia
PCPAP	periodic CPAP
PDP	personal development plan
PE	pulmonary embolus
PEEP	positive end expiratory pressure
PEFR	peak expiratory flow rate
PEP	positive expiratory pressure
pH	negative logarithm of hydrogen ion concentration in moles per litre
PICU	paediatric intensive care unit
PIP	positive inspiratory pressure
Plt	platelets
PMH	past medical history
p.r.n.	'as required'
PS	pressure support *or* pulmonary stenosis
PVC	premature ventricular contraction

RLL	right lower lobe
RML	right middle lobe
RR	respiratory rate
RS	respiratory system
RTA	road traffic accident
RUL	right upper lobe

SAH	subarachnoid haemorrhage
SaO$_2$	saturation of oxygen in arterial blood (shown in ABGs)
SB	spina bifida
SH	social history
SIRS	systemic inflammatory response
SMA	spinal muscular atrophy
SOB	shortness of breath
SOBAR	shortness of breath at rest
SOBOE	shortness of breath on exertion
SpO$_2$	pulse oximetry arterial oxygen saturation
SVCO	superior vena cava obstruction
SWOT	strengths, weaknesses, opportunities, threats
TB	tuberculosis
TEE	thoracic expansion exercises
TENS	transcutaneous electrical nerve stimulation
TGA	transposition of great arteries
TMR	transmyocardial revascularization
TOF	tetralogy of Fallot
TV	tidal volume
UZ	upper zone
VAS	visual analogue scale
V/Q	ventilation/perfusion ratio
VC	vital capacity
VSD	ventricular septal defect
WCC	white cell count
WOB	work of breathing

Index